CLEMENS VON PIRQUET
His Life and Work

CLEMENS VON PIRQUET
HIS LIFE AND WORK

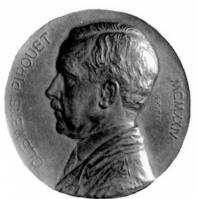

Medal of von Pirquet struck
on the occasion of his fiftieth birthday
and presented by his assistants
in the Vienna *Kinderklinik*.

BY RICHARD WAGNER, M.D.

The Johns Hopkins Press
Baltimore, Maryland

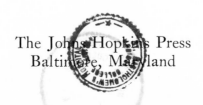

M4472
25/7/80

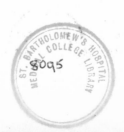

DEDICATED

To all the students
of the *Kinderklinik*,
University of Vienna

Foreword

Through his life and his work Clemens von Pirquet fulfilled the fondest dream of any children's doctor: to be a pioneer in unknown fields, a physician giving the finest treatment to his patients, and a benefactor to all mankind. His tuberculin test and other skin tests are applied daily all over the world, and his theory of allergy throws light on a great many pathological phenomena. Such branches of medicine as immunology, biometrics, biostatistics, and social pediatrics have developed in large part from the stimulus of his work. He pioneered in founding modern pediatrics and biological medicine.

Clemens von Pirquet was one of those remarkable masters of the Vienna School who personified the research and teaching of medicine during a glorious period. In his appearance, his manners, and his thought he was an aristocrat throughout a life which was wracked by the dramas of European history and ended in personal and family tragedy. Those who had the honor to know him retain a profound memory which calls to mind certain illustrious men of the Renaissance whose knowledge was universal. Von Pirquet knew several languages; he spoke both French and English like his native tongue. His was a broad scientific, artistic, and literary culture.

Von Pirquet taught pediatrics in America and was as happy in the literary worlds of France and Great Britain as he had been in the Germany of the past. His ancestors came from Belgium and later settled in Austria. He was trained to philosophical thought as a student at the University of Louvain. He was the spiritual son of the whole of western Europe. His was a generation of generous hopes, great ideas, and fundamental discoveries—then heartbreak and ruin. His memory evokes above all a man who, having achieved fame and the admiration of his contemporaries in every country, found comfort from the disaster and grief of the world by dedicating himself to the children of mankind until, before the approach of yet more fearful horrors, he quit life abruptly.

He worked in his chosen field with passion, concentrating on the effort to understand the biological facts which he studied minutely, seeking a doctrine which could enrich the phenomena that his reasoning and his essays on human beings brought to light. His works on revaccination, on the sensitivity of the skin to tuberculin, and on nutrition are models of analysis and synthesis. When his views were contested he first fought back, then he came to the conclusion that if his ideas were not accepted at once, at least when they did triumph they would be considered as original.

The United States will remember that he was the first professor of pediatrics at The Johns Hopkins University in Baltimore; France, that he brought to the Pediatric Society in Paris the discovery of the tuberculin test; Great Britain, that he joined with his colleagues of the British Medical Association in the first effort to prevent tuberculosis in young children; and the whole world, that he was the force behind the *Union Internationale de Sécours aux Enfants,* established at Geneva, and chairman of the Committee for Child Hygiene at the League of Nations. As France's representative on the Committee for Child Hygiene, I was impressed by von Pirquet's ability to organize and to visualize the importance of pediatrics and the social sciences.

Von Pirquet proved his genius as a scientist while still very young. He was only twenty-nine when he presented to the Imperial Academy of Sciences in Vienna a paper on the theory of infectious diseases. From that moment he became one of the most prominent investigators of the European research team which created immunology, a basic discipline dedicated to the study of the conflict between the antigen and its host.

In Vienna, at the pediatric clinic which he organized, he established the greatest school of pediatrics of the time. He was helped in his work by his disciples Bela Schick—deservedly the best known—Nobel, Wagner, Mayerhofer, and v. Gröer. As he himself declared near the end of his life, he had been able to see the impact of his personal ideas on the scientific world. Von Pirquet and his followers, instead of experimenting on animals, gave clinicians the example of work carried on directly on man and child in order that sick children might be better understood and cured at the same time.

Being myself one of the rare survivors of that past, I can still see his handsome profile, his tall stature, his strikingly bright blue eyes, and his fine features which expressed so much charm and kindness when he greeted me in his clinic or came to my home, together with Madame von Pirquet, to meet the French doctors eager to honor him. He took pleasure in showing his clinic with its modern fittings, its devices for protection against the hospital infections then so much feared, the veranda for small tuberculous patients, the school for convalescents. He lived there surrounded by deferential affection. His natural simplicity was striking in a man so universally acclaimed. Invited to an international meeting in London (where we met for the first time) and greeted by Sir Neville Chamberlain (then Minister of Health), Clemens von Pirquet with a charming sense of modesty tried to remain in the background. He had to be forced to accept the first place, one which he has kept among the leaders of modern pediatrics.

ROBERT DEBRÉ

L'Académie des Sciences, Paris

Acknowledgments

The author wishes to express his gratitude to the John Simon Guggenheim Foundation, New York City; the National Library of Medicine, National Institutes of Health, Bethesda, Maryland; and the Charles H. Hood Dairy Foundation, Charlestown, Massachusetts, for their generous support of the research upon which this biography is based. The courtesy extended by John B. Blake, Ph.D., Chief of the History of Medicine Division, National Library of Medicine, Bethesda, and by Monsieur P. J.-M. Carvin, Chief of Communications and Dossiers of the Archives of the Health Section of the League of Nations, World Health Organization, Geneva, Switzerland, in granting ready access to the resources of their libraries, greatly aided the substantiation of data.

Grateful thanks are herewith given to Dame Harriette Chick for her sustained interest, to Miss E. M. M. Hume for reading portions of the manuscript and offering suggestions, to Miss Mary Corcoran for her careful revision and editing of the text, and to Mrs. Doris H. Carlin for typing the manuscript.

Contents

Illustrations

Figures

Introduction

The aim of this historical study is twofold: to present a biographical sketch of Clemens von Pirquet, and to evaluate the significance of his scientific discoveries and their influence on present-day thinking in medicine. Writing biography is a delicate matter. A biographer may unconsciously reveal too much about himself at the expense of his subject or he may distort the truth through the manner in which facts and anecdotes are arranged or omitted. In a medical biography, technicalities are not entirely avoidable. An attempt will be made to satisfy physicians, as well as other scientists and the general reader. Students of medical history may benefit from knowing the explorers of dark, unknown areas, the leaders of a period, and the driving forces that changed the concepts of medicine through the fertility of new ideas.

Biography of scientists is complicated by the problem of making the technical achievements of the subject understandable to the lay reader. Because of this, lives of scientists are usually written by other scientists, the result too often being not biography, but a laboratory report on a specimen that seems never to have been alive.[1]

From daily contacts with medical students in the United States this biographer has become aware of the striking fact that von Pirquet's name is almost unknown, although he died only thirty-eight years ago. The concept of allergy and the von Pirquet tuberculin test are taken for granted and the name of their discoverer is no longer attached to them. Perhaps this is a sign of real greatness. Meanwhile, allergy has become an independent branch of medicine in this country, and the tuberculin test is routinely carried out on each patient admitted to every children's hospital. Few of von Pirquet's co-workers are still alive. Therefore, it seems urgent to bring to life all of his genius, that posterity may remember and appreciate him for what he was. This book aims to present his work and to correlate it with the different periods of his life, rather than merely to chronicle his achieve-

[1] Harold J. Sharlin, *Bull. Atomic Scientists* (November, 1963), p. 27.

ments. "The biographer must rather seek to understand the personality, to integrate personality with achievement, and to interpret the result for its meaning to general history."[2] Biographical sections will include what is considered important, illuminating, or interesting in the life history of this man of genius, without intruding too far into his privacy. However, for the sake of revealing the truth, his privacy cannot be kept entirely inviolate, since it seems important to analyze and understand the character of a man who committed suicide at the summit of a successful life. In contrast to the frequent practice of idealizing the subject of a biography and repeatedly emphasizing his greatness, in this study von Pirquet's weaknesses will be considered as important to an analysis of his genius as his exploits.

The ten years from 1919 until 1929 constituted the period in which, through daily contact in professional and private life, the biographer had the opportunity to study the personality of Clemens von Pirquet. That association is the justification for writing his biography. In addition to personal observations, this study drew upon papers and communications supplied by members of the von Pirquet family, records of The Johns Hopkins Hospital, and von Pirquet's own conversations and published works. Many documents which could have provided supplemental data were destroyed when the *Kinderklinik* was bombed during World War II.

What is so outstanding in this man? What made him different from other famous pioneers in science and medicine? In spite of being trained in the classical tradition of the Vienna School of Medicine, with emphasis on diagnosis and pathological anatomy, he never excelled in these aspects of medical science. Although a keen observer, he had no desire to study individual, so-called "interesting," cases. His interest was centered chiefly on the general, unsolved problems in medicine, including infectious diseases; serum sickness and vaccination, which led to the concept of allergy; tuberculosis, culminating in the discovery of the von Pirquet test; nutrition; anthropometrics; graphic and statistical analysis of growth and development; vital statistics; seasonal incidence of disease; and preventive medicine, particularly as it related to nutritional deficiencies.

[2] *Ibid.*

We might say that in von Pirquet's time medicine was at the threshold of a new era, characterized by the development and application of discoveries in other sciences and by X-ray techniques, and that intuition, memory, and empiricism were being replaced by more exact data. This did not preclude the value of experience or of diagnostic flair, but widened the base upon which medicine rested. These years at the beginning of the twentieth century, during which von Pirquet pioneered, marked the transition of medicine from an art to a science. Von Pirquet was no longer a clinician of the old school, but a scientist through and through. With lightning flashes of insight he clarified hitherto unexplored areas. It is no wonder that occasionally he met opposition and criticism. When the clinician leaves the problems of disease and trespasses into a more comprehensive neighboring field, he is accompanied by the secret fears of those he leaves behind and is received with mistrust by those he approaches. He runs the double risk of losing the former group and of gaining little from the latter. It has been thus with the exploring physicians of all times.

Cambridge, Massachusetts
March 17, 1967

Chronological Table

May 12, 1874	Born in Hirschstetten, near Vienna
1880–84	Educated at home with private teacher
1884–87	Attended *Schottengymnasium*, a school staffed by members of the Benedictine Order
1887–92	Studied at a Jesuit boarding school in Kalksburg, near Vienna
1892	Passed matriculation examination with honors at the *Theresianum*
1892–93	Studied theology at University of Innsbruck, Tyrol, Austria
1893–94	Studied philosophy at University of Louvain, Belgium
1894	Ph.B., University of Louvain
1895	University of Vienna
1896–97	University of Königsberg, Prussia
1897–1900	University of Graz
1900	M.D., University of Graz Six months as medical officer in the armed forces; then started pediatric training in Berlin under Otto von Heubner
1901–02	Internship and residency at *Universitäts Kinderklinik* under Theodor Escherich
1903–09	Clinical assistant at the *Kinderklinik*
1904	Married Maria Christine van Husen
1908	*Privatdozent* (university lecturer) of pediatrics
1909	Professor of Pediatrics, The Johns Hopkins University, Baltimore
1910	Professor of Pediatrics, University of Breslau
1911–29	Professor of Pediatrics, University of Vienna
February 28, 1929	Death by suicide

CLEMENS VON PIRQUET
His Life and Work

I

Auspicious Beginnings

The fourth son in his family, Clemens von Pirquet was born on
May 12, 1874, in Hirschstetten, near Vienna. There his father,
Peter Zeno Freiherr (Baron) von Pirquet, owned an estate
famous for its tree nursery. Besides three older brothers, Theodor,
Peter, and Silverio, Clemens had one younger brother, Guido, and
two older sisters, Agnes and Margarete.

His paternal ancestors came from Belgium, which until the
Battle of Waterloo in 1815 had been an Austrian province. Over
a long period of time they had lived in Liège. Originally the sur-
name was Mardaga, but at the end of the seventeenth century
one ancestor, for purposes of inheritance, assumed the name
Pirquet dit Mardaga. The members of the family were patricians
of high repute who were active in such professions as the law,
commerce, or the army. At the time of the French Revolution
the great grandfather, Jean Martin Auguste Pirquet dit Mardaga,
was commander of the bodyguard for the Prince Archbishop of
Méan. After Liège was captured by the French revolution-
ary army in 1794, Jean Martin Auguste was left destitute with
eleven children to raise. However, befriended by neighboring
families, the children were adequately brought up and educated.
One son, Pierre Lambert Auguste Pirquet dit Mardaga, a great-
uncle of Clemens, joined the Belgian regiment Beaulieu, which
remained faithful to Austria. His younger brother, Pierre Martin,
who became the grandfather of Clemens, joined the same regiment in 1799 and both brothers were on active service throughout
the Napoleonic wars. When Ebelsberg was taken by storm on
May 9, 1809, Pierre Martin so distinguished himself that he was
awarded his country's highest decoration, the Order of the Empress Maria Theresa, for exceeding bravery. In May 1815, for
courage before the enemy at a surprise attack on Cesenatico in
Italy, he was decorated with the Order of the Emperor Leopold,
and in 1818 the title of Baronet of Cesenatico was bestowed upon
him. During the years from 1820 to 1830 he led with great suc-

cess a raiding party in Istria and the littoral, mopping up bands of brigands who had infested that area. In the last years of his life he served as lieutenant colonel in the bodyguard (*Arcieren Leibgarde*) of the Austrian Emperor, a distinguished honor. After a long and full life he died in 1861.[1]

The many descendants of Baronet Pierre Martin Pirquet dit Mardaga stemmed from his marriage in 1825 to Johanna Freiin (Baroness) von Mayern. They had four children: Anton, also awarded the Order of the Empress Maria Theresa and subsequently killed at the Battle of Rivoli in 1848; Marie, wife of Captain Guido Freiherr von Eiselsberg, whose son Anton became the famous surgeon at the University of Vienna; Jennie, a nun in the Order of the Sacred Heart; and Peter Zeno, father of Clemens. Thus Clemens Freiherr von Pirquet was a member of the third generation of the family in Austria. Peter Zeno acquired an estate in Hirschstetten, near the historic battlefield of Aspern, in 1868. During World War II it was badly damaged by bombing, and later the estate was sold to a religious order. The building called *Ziegelhof*, which Clemens had restored and used as his country home, was completely destroyed.

Clemens' father played an important part in the Austrian parliament as a representative of the landowners party. Later he became chairman of a parliamentary group called Friends of Peace of Austria. His ideas on agriculture seem to have been akin to those later evident in the brilliant mind of his son. Among the father's hobbies were graphic analysis, chart-making, and statistical studies; his son had similar tastes. Peter Zeno became interested in educational reforms in the high schools and universities, and expressed his ideas in a letter to Theodor Billroth, surgeon at the University of Vienna. Clemens' father was a gifted poet and also tried his hand as a playwright. A little poem of baroque flavor, which he wrote to honor the administrative director of the estate on his nameday was recited by Clemens when he was three years and ten months old. One of Peter Zeno's plays was submitted for performance in the State Theater of Vienna. He died in 1906.

Clemens' mother, Flora Freiin von Pereira-Arnstein, came from a Vienna court banker's family of Sephardic descent. Her

---

[1] A biography of this remarkable man was written by P. Hanquet: Société de l'Ordre de Léopold. *Compte Rendu de l'Assemblée Générale Statutaire*, May, 1959.

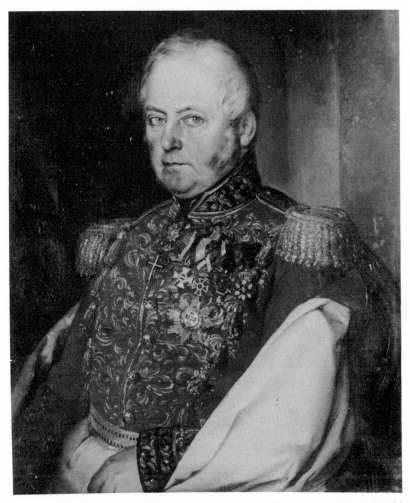

Peter Martin Pirquet, grandfather of Clemens, in his uniform as lieutenant colonel in the bodyguard of the Austrian Emperor.

family's salon was an attractive center of fashionable society, especially during the Congress of Vienna in 1815. She was a devout Catholic and her religious fervor was largely influential in Clemens' early decision to study theology. In the tradition of the Austrian nobility, the eldest son succeeded his father as the landed proprietor. One of the younger sons might become an officer in the army or navy, another might enter the diplomatic service, and one was usually destined for the Church. The property was thus kept intact and transmitted from generation to generation through the first-born son. Contrary to custom, after the death of Flora von Pirquet in 1912 the rights in the Pirquet estate were divided equally among the seven children. One of the sons, Silverio, became the *Pächter* or landholder, thus in a sense keeping the property together. This arrangement appears to have led to disagreement among the heirs and to a family lawsuit which was still unsettled at the end of Clemens von Pirquet's life.

During his childhood the family lived year-round in the country, without luxury or pretension but comfortably and in the security of the late nineteenth century. Clemens spent his first years in the care of nursemaids. According to his older brother Silverio, he was late in beginning to talk and was shy during early childhood. However, a letter written to his mother before he was five years old has been preserved and is noteworthy both in its clarity and in his expression of deep affection. The handwriting consisted of carefully drawn German characters, which were taught to children in grammar school before the Latin alphabet. By the age of six, Clemens seems to have become quite active and courageous. In her diary[2] his mother dedicated to him a little poem, "The Brave Hero," listing a variety of heroic deeds associated particularly with pony rides and dog fights. When Clemens was seven years old he played with a group of boys who lived nearby, and Silverio described him as the leader of the gang. One of his best friends was the son of the village blacksmith. A photograph taken at this time shows the von Pirquet children with their parents prior to a family outing. From numerous entries in the diary one can recognize the mother's strong influence in the upbringing of her children, their dependence upon her, and their mutual attachment. A great many entries concern Clemens, of whom she seems to have been particularly fond. The diary also conspicuously reflects her ideology. Pages and pages are filled with religious meditations and the exact dates of her Holy Communions. Clemens was ten when he made his first confession.

A private teacher gave careful elementary instruction to all seven children at home. When the von Pirquet sons were ready to enter the gymnasium, in which they were to receive preparation for university study, their parents took an apartment in Vienna and Clemens attended the first three grades in the *Schot-*

[2] I am greatly indebted to Dr. Agnes Sorgo, a niece of von Pirquet, for permission to refer to the diary.

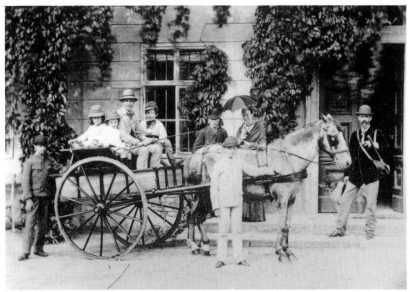

The von Pirquet parents and children at Hirschstetten.
Clemens is standing in the center foreground.

tengymnasium, called the "Eton of Austria." Johann Strauss and
the last Emperor of Austria, Karl I, were educated there. Clemens' last five years of gymnasium were spent in a Jesuit boarding
school in Kalksburg, near Vienna. He was on the honor roll of his
class every year, and the great delight of his mother in his achievements can be seen by the entries in her diary. The Jesuit priests,
who were interested in the future vocations of their pupils, considered him a good candidate for the priesthood and supported
the idea to the satisfaction of his extremely pious mother. After
passing the matriculation examination with honors at the *Theresi-
anum*[3] in 1892, he studied theology at the University of Innsbruck
in Austria (1892–93) and philosophy at the University of Louvain
in Belgium (1893–94), where he gained a bachelor's degree (Ph.B).
His more worldly father advised him to register not only with the
theological faculty but also with the law school, to keep open a
line of retreat in case Clemens should change his mind concerning
his vocation. His cousin (later his brother-in-law), Anton von
Eiselsberg, with whom Clemens discussed his plans to become a
priest, considered him too immature and warned against a hasty

[3] Founded by Empress Maria Theresa to educate the sons of the nobility.

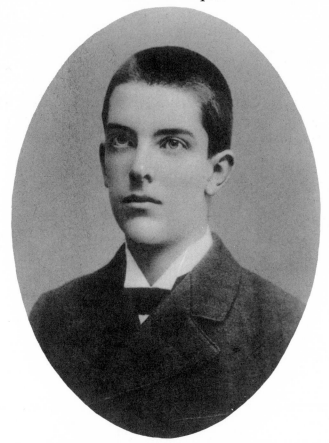

Clemens von Pirquet at the age of eighteen.

decision. During his second term at Louvain he participated in a pilgrimage to Lourdes which seems to have precipitated an emotional crisis. He decided to give up his religious studies, although he always remained a Catholic. His brother recalled that the decision to quit theology caused his mother keen disappointment.[4]

In his subsequent determination to enter medicine, as in his unconventional marriage, von Pirquet also disappointed his family. By the standards of the Austrian nobility, medicine was not an entirely acceptable profession. Even in the military hier-

[4] In Charles Darwin's life the situation was reversed. Since Darwin did not wish to be a physician, his father proposed that he become a clergyman. "Nor was this intention and my father's wish ever formally given up, but died a natural death when on leaving Cambridge I joined the *Beagle* as a naturalist" (*The Autobiography of Charles R. Darwin* [London: Collins, 1958], p. 57).

archy of the Habsburg Empire the doctor was not held in high
regard; his rank in the cavalry was close to that of the veterinar-
ian. After World War I the attitude toward medicine was
modified greatly, and three of von Pirquet's nephews and nieces
became physicians. The motive which prompted him to study
medicine is obscure. His decision was probably not influenced
directly by his brother-in-law, in spite of their friendship, but
was rather a protest against the oversolicitude of his mother.

Little information is available about von Pirquet's student
days in Innsbruck and Louvain. His mother's diary ceased in
1892. However, he once jokingly remarked to this biographer
that part of his duties while a student at the University of Innsbruck consisted in visiting prostitutes in the neighborhood—we
assume for the purpose of converting them. Soon after he left
Louvain he began to study medicine.

It was customary in nineteenth-century Europe for medical
students to move from one university to another. A valuable
aspect of medical education was the opportunity to observe a
professor's techniques and his approach to clinical problems. From
attendance at lectures the student gained a great deal of wisdom
which was not published in any textbook. On the other hand, he
was under less pressure than the American medical student, who
receives superior training along the lines of generally accepted
textbook material. In Europe a closer rapport often existed
between the head of a department and his students, and young
men were eager to be associated with outstanding professors in
the various disciplines. Thus it was not unusual that von Pirquet
should have attended three medical schools for study in the
departments for which each was noted. His first year was spent
at the University of Vienna, which had many outstanding faculty
members. Pathology was taught by Weichselbaum, who discovered the organism responsible for cerebrospinal meningitis.
Autopsies were performed on every patient who died in the hospital, and it was largely because of pathology and brilliant diagnosis
that the Vienna School of Medicine became famous. Weichselbaum's fine teaching, plus the wealth of pathological material,
made his courses extremely popular, and there was never an
empty seat at his lectures. Hermann Widerhofer then held the
chair of pediatrics, Ebner taught microscopic anatomy, Exner
headed the department of physiology, and Nothnagel, who had
come from Germany, taught internal medicine. Von Pirquet once

said that the instruction which he received in nutrition was use-
less. Instead of discussing dietary requirements, Nothnagel told
the students which wines should be prescribed to stimulate a
patient "and he almost gave their vintage."

The next two terms were spent at the University of Königsberg
in East Prussia. At that time Anton von Eiselsberg held the
chair of surgery at Königsberg, and the presence of his brother-in-
law may have influenced von Pirquet's choice of a university. He
attended Professor von Eiselsberg's lectures in surgery. One of
the most popular of the preclinical sciences was physiology, which
was taught by Professor Hermann. Von Pirquet learned research
methods in the physiology laboratory and carried out his first investigations there.

In his autobiography, von Eiselsberg mentions hiking and
sledding with Clemens in the Samland near Königsberg.[5] Because
of the biting cold, this activity must have been strenuous. When
asked about Clemens' progress, von Eiselsberg declared that he
had never had such a lazy pupil. Years afterward, von Pirquet
mentioned that he had fallen asleep in one of von Eiselsberg's
lectures, an incident which was never forgotten nor forgiven.
Throughout his life he maintained an aloof attitude toward
surgery. Even when he was in charge of the Vienna *Kinderklinik*
he did not maintain a surgical service there. Children with problems suggesting such treatment were seen in consultation with a
competent surgeon and, if surgery was considered necessary, were
transferred to the university surgical clinic. Von Pirquet was
afraid that his nurses would lose interest in medical pediatric care
if they were to become familiar with the more dramatic service on
a surgical ward or, as he liked to say, "if they should smell blood."

Von Pirquet continued his medical studies at the University
of Graz, where Theodor Escherich was professor of pediatrics, and
gained his M.D. degree there in 1900. He was always an honor
student. When time permitted, he engaged in active mountain
climbing in company with his friend Haberer, who afterward
became professor of surgery in Cologne. Later in life von Pirquet
lost his enthusiasm for this sport. He questioned the pleasure and
satisfaction to be derived from climbing mountains and even
frowned when his assistants participated in such activity; a
mountain became to him merely a heap of stone.

[5] Anton v. Eiselsberg, *Lebensweg eines Chirurgen* (Innsbruck: Tyrolia Verlag,
1937).

For some time he entertained the idea of becoming a psychiatrist, and one can only speculate about his reasons for abandoning that plan. Psychiatry was then mainly descriptive, with a strong tendency to relate certain psychiatric entities to organic changes. Men like Charcot, Bernheim, Kräpelin, Forel, and Bleuler were representative of the period. Freud's new doctrines were frequently ridiculed, and serious discussion of psychoanalysis took place only in a small circle around the master. More nonmedical people attended his lectures than students of medicine. Von Pirquet was never heard to make a remark hostile to psychoanalysis, even though the new psychology had already penetrated not only psychiatry but also various other areas within the *Geisteswissenschaften*, including the social sciences, art, religion, education, and even the courtroom.

In retrospect, it is easy to understand why a scholar of von Pirquet's caliber and temperament was not attracted by psychiatry. His methods of thought and those of the psychiatrists were entirely different, like straight lines in different planes which never meet. Nevertheless, all his life he retained an interest in the subject.

The complex problem which faces a young physician who decides to specialize must be visualized apart from external factors, such as the chance offer of a position at the right time, or family considerations. The layman's idea that pediatrics is chosen as a specialty because the individual is particularly fond of children is too superficial to explain von Pirquet's choice. To enjoy the presence of children, to watch their play, to listen to their songs, to see them in constant, lively motion, and to seek to understand them gives the satisfaction derived from observing the youthful zest of any living being.

None of these interests provided sufficient motivation for von Pirquet's choice of pediatrics as his specialty. Kindness to children and to people in general is a minimum requirement for dealing successfully with human beings; kindness was part of von Pirquet's nature. Nothnagel, one of the great medical leaders of that time, used to say: "Only a kind person can be a good physician." That sentiment is appealing, especially to the patient, but kindness is not the only attribute needed by the physician. Von Pirquet's scholarly, brilliant mind sought other satisfactions. His overwhelming urge was to become a scientist. That urge gained power from an irresistible desire to explore, to find the truth, to clarify hitherto inexplicable phenomena by keen observation, to analyze the apparently complicated and reduce it to simplicity, and to replace cumbersome descriptive details by formulae. At that time such a special form of scientific interest could find suitable expression in pediatrics.

During the early years of his medical career, bacteriology, serology, and immunology were emerging sciences which attracted gifted, promising students. Young physicians who were not in a hurry to start general practice and aspired to an academic career could work in a laboratory as well as attend to their clinical duties. Depending upon preference and interest, the choice might be pathology, bacteriology and immunology, biochemistry, or pharmacology. In many instances successful laboratory studies opened the door to an academic career for a clinical assistant. Von Pirquet's keen interest in infectious diseases, which are predominant in childhood, was obviously the factor which led him into pediatrics. In the latter part of the nineteenth and the early twentieth centuries, the most important aspects of child care were control of infectious disease and nutritional disorders. His first fundamental discoveries resulted from careful clinical studies—daily observation and recording of the character and time factor in the response of individuals to the administration of smallpox vaccine or the foreign protein in horse serum. From those observations his ideas on incubation time and allergy were formulated. Like Gregor Mendel, who in solitude came to far-reaching conclusions and laid the cornerstone of the science of genetics, Clemens von Pirquet changed the concepts of immunology by applying the same methods of simple experimentation, careful observation, and numerical evaluation of results.

Through an unusually favorable combination of circumstances—including patrician ancestors of exceptional intelligence, an excellent education, and a distinctive creativity—Clemens von Pirquet became not only an outstanding physician and scientist but also a renowned humanitarian. His early studies in theology and philosophy, although not pursued to completion, nevertheless influenced his decision to enter the field of medicine. The course of medicine was advanced by this choice and by another critical decision which shaped his life—namely, whether to accept a distinguished invitation from Emile Roux to become a member of the Pasteur Institute in Paris or an almost simultaneous offer from The Johns Hopkins University in Baltimore.

II

Personality of a Genius

The final structure of a personality results from the integration of environmental and intrinsic factors. Family, education, religion, social relations, customs, the not-easily-definable atmosphere in which an individual is brought up, and the historical and political situation in his native country all exert strong influences on the formation of his personality. Some intrinsic factors are genetically conditioned but can be modified by developmental and environmental influences. An attempt will be made to interpret the latter concept in evaluating von Pirquet's personality.

Although national characteristics change but little, each period of history creates a specific atmosphere. To assume that this atmosphere influences any individual living in the period may be a superficial and too general conclusion. Vienna, the capital of the Habsburg Empire during the formative years of von Pirquet's life, was and is still considered the city of happy-go-lucky folk on the Blue Danube who in the evening at garden restaurants in the Vienna woods taste the new wine, singing and indulging in a swaying, sweet, frothy frivolity. That generalization is just as absurd as to characterize the French mind as always abnormally preoccupied with matters of sex. The famous Viennese *Gemütlichkeit* has been condemned as a form of self-indulgence which was intended to avoid sharp conflicts and strong convictions and served as a mechanism for escape from reality. It is true that the Viennese, young and old alike, were extremely interested in the theater, not only in plays but also in actors and actresses and their private lives. Yet such a preoccupation is no different from the American interest in movie and television stars, the Beatles, or heroes of sport.

There was, however, another Austria, a center of art, learning, and science from which radiated powerful cultural influences. Vienna, for instance, exerted a considerable influence on the development of medicine in the United States and throughout the world. Austria at the end of the nineteenth and the beginning of the twentieth centuries was the Austria of Mach and Boltzman in physics, of Billroth in surgery, of Bruckner and Mahler in music, of Rilke, Kafka, and Kraus in literature, of Kokoschka in portrait painting, of Freud in the new psychology, and of Clemens von Pirquet in pediatrics.

Born and brought up in the peaceful years before World Wars I and II, von Pirquet was a product of that period even though he differed in many respects from his contemporaries, particularly other professors. He also differed markedly in his ability to project beyond his own era. In the mind of the public, an idealized image of the university professor had evolved. He was expected to be not only a great scholar and scientist, a top teacher and lecturer—and in medicine a top physician—but also to have a unique and warm personality, to be an idealist (not interested in money-making), and a man who contributed to the cultural and artistic life of his time. A few mannerisms and idiosyncrasies were excused and even cherished. Ordinary pleasures were thought to be inconsistent with such a person's way of life. To characterize this kind of personality the German language has a specific term, *Prachtmensch*, meaning a man akin to the Renaissance type. In appearance these men were different from businessmen, executives, bank managers, statesmen, or diplomats, and adopted many of the externals of artists. Long beards, hats with wide brims, velvet jackets, or unconventional neckties were characteristic. Even to look somewhat unkempt was acceptable. Needless to say, the great men's pupils often imitated the master's dress and his mannerisms. If the pupils were not intellectually superior, theirs was usually a hollow mimicry. To quote Schiller: "How he hawks and spits, indeed, I may say, you have copied and caught in the cleverest way."

Von Pirquet's appearance, unlike the professorial image, was always that of a gentleman. He dressed carefully and wore conservative clothes. He talked in simple language without affectation or mannerisms, had a good sense of humor, and was fond of such ordinary pleasures as a game of bridge, a good joke, a dance, a glass of wine. He was not afraid to be as other men because of his own strong and distinguished personality. He was considerate of others, yet not afraid to be outspoken when the situation warranted. In one instance a manufacturer had placed von Pirquet's name on the label of a nationally known baby food to imply an endorsement of the product. Von Pirquet had not given permission for use of his name and asked the head of the firm to come to his office and explain. In an attempt to justify himself the manufacturer presented his arguments at great length. Finally von Pirquet stood up and concluded the conversation abruptly with the remark: "You know what? I don't like your face."

From my own professional association with him, of ten years' duration, I conclude that he had enough self-assurance so that he felt he could afford not to know everything about his own field. I recall that when he was lecturing on some problem with which he did not feel perfectly familiar he would call upon one of his assistants who had specialized training to discuss the problem while he himself sat on a front bench and listened. It did not occur to him to bother about prestige or protocol. During rounds, when he was asked for his opinion on an undiagnosed case, he used to say with tongue in cheek: "*Kraft meines Amtes entscheide ich*" (ex officio I decide).

That the omniscience expected of the German professor was alien to him was illustrated in the last serious discussion I had with him, approximately ten days before his suicide. I had been talking with Wenkebach, professor of medicine, about a patient in whom he was interested. He asked me to give a message to von Pirquet in which he sharply criticized a recent postgraduate course of the medical faculty as inadequate, in contrast to the previous course which he felt served as a better model. When I returned to the *Kinderklinik* von Pirquet was sitting at his table, lost in such deep concentration that I was reluctant to disturb him. In those final days he was applying the finishing touches to his book, *Allergy of the Life Phases*. He must have been in a hurry, since the date of the suicide was undoubtedly fixed. When he finally became aware of my presence, I gave him the message. As he listened he recalled himself, looking at me as though from another world. Then he said: "There is one thing which will not be said about me after my death—that I was a 'German professor.' " The meaning became obvious retrospectively to one who had known him well. The German professor was to him the personification of a man who, because of his position in society, was expected to assume the heavy burden of educating the younger generation and of improving the world. Von Pirquet knew his own limitations and did not regard himself as one of the chosen leaders of mankind. In fact, he used to make fun of people whose ability was not adequate to their position, saying *"wem Gott ein Amt gegeben, dem gibt er auch den Verstand"* (to him on whom God bestowed an office, he also gave a brain).

Simplicity, open-mindedness, and a matter-of-fact attitude were outstanding features of von Pirquet's personality. They were clearly manifested when he was called in consultation to see a private patient. At that time, an eminent physician was thought to be above an interest in making money—an attitude prevalent in a society with a tendency toward insincerity and hypocrisy. The fee would be placed in an envelope and given to the doctor in such a way that not even those in the immediate vicinity could see that he was being paid. Von Pirquet was straightforward and felt no shyness in accepting a well-deserved fee. He would unconcernedly open the envelope and count the bills in the presence of his patient.

Late in his life, on his estate at Hirschstetten, he founded the first dairy in Austria to produce pasteurized and certified milk for infants. At that time I was working with him on important experiments to enrich milk with the antirachitic factor by irradiating the cows with ultraviolet light or giving them large doses of cod-liver oil. To maintain an adequate supply of milk it was necessary from time to time to replace a cow. One day von Pirquet was summoned to Hungary to see the child of a prince in consultation. When he came back and was asked how he had fared, he smiled and said: "It was fine, worth half a cow." That was his monetary unit just then.

People who worked for him or for the clinic were always paid for their services, even when they were of a clerical or routine nature, although this was not always the practice in similar institutions. He did not believe in the efficiency of volunteer workers, knowing too well that after a short initial period of enthusiasm their efforts usually slackened. When I was appointed at the *Kinderklinik* the youngest assistant was unpaid, but von Pirquet immediately provided a fellowship equal to the salary of an assistant. He advanced the first installment of my salary from his own wallet, since official regulations delayed payment of the fellowship. Von Pirquet's attitude in all matters regarding money was a significant component of his character. It seemed to be an unconscious protest against any kind of insincerity or injustice.

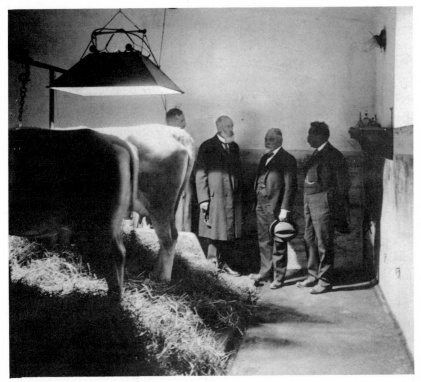

Visitors to the dairy barn at Hirschstetten, where an experiment was being carried on to enrich milk with vitamin D. Von Pirquet, at extreme left, is standing beside Hainisch, President of the Austrian Republic.

An analysis of the character of Clemens von Pirquet reveals the distinctive quality of genius. Many definitions have been proposed in an attempt to explain what it is that makes an individual a genius—different from other members of *Homo sapiens* —but none is exhaustive enough to characterize the entire class. Interpretations have been offered by philosophers and psychiatrists. The German psychiatrist Kretschmer devoted a significant monograph to the problem in which he underscored the relation of genius to psychopathology. Kretschmer also associated certain somatotypes with specific forms of insanity—the leptosome type with schizophrenia, the pyknic or eurosome type with manic-depressive psychosis. Even among normal types, Kretschmer pursued the antithesis of psychic behavior patterns and distinguished between schizothymic and cyclothymic personalities. Exact logicians and systematic individuals belong to the schizothymic group. In Kretschmer's nomenclature, von Pirquet was a leptosome somatotype.[1] The Italian physician and criminologist Lombroso pointed out the familiar association of genius and insanity. Long before Lombroso and Kretschmer, Schopenhauer said in his dry way: "The genius is nearer to insanity than to average intelligence." Even in antiquity, Seneca declared: *"Non est magnum ingenium sine mixtura dementiae."*

Since von Pirquet's life ended in suicide, that approach is tempting. Freud, however, considered that pathographies or medical studies of the morbid conditions affecting various famous personages were of very little value in throwing light on their personalities and consequently on their work. Here, a more or less descriptive approach will be followed. Anecdotes and attitudes which I remember may occasionally illustrate and characterize best what was outstanding and unusual in Clemens von Pirquet.

Genius seems to be a biological entity, a plus variation, established in the specific architectonics of the brain. In favor of that assumption is the linkage of certain characteristics in the same person, such as the gifts for music and mathematics. Familial inheritance of genius is occasionally encountered, as was shown by Galton; it occurred in von Pirquet's family. His younger brother, Guido, was a keen mathematician and physicist with a degree in engineering. Long before such ideas were looked upon seriously, he visualized a method by which space travel could be accomplished. His concepts were originally brushed aside as fantastic; only after World War II were they recognized and honored.

One characteristic of a genius is the intuitive association of his discoveries or observations with other phenomena, not always obviously related, and the immediate anticipation of all the consequences of the discovery. In von Pirquet's preliminary report on the theory of infectious diseases, which he deposited with the Imperial Academy of Sciences in Vienna in 1903, he had anticipated the conclusions from simple yet careful observation and analysis. He had realized from the first that the causative organism is not primarily responsible for the signs and symptoms manifest in many of the infectious diseases. The characteristic signs of the disease result rather from the production of antibodies by the host which has been invaded and from their interaction with

[1] E. Kretschmer, *Geniale Menschen* (Berlin: Julius Springer, 1929).

the invading organisms. In the same way, he realized that the proteins of injected horse serum do not directly cause the signs of serum sickness. It is only after antibodies to the horse-serum proteins have been formed that the antigen-antibody complex produces serum sickness.

Another genius, Claude Bernard, who discovered a starch-like substance in the liver called glycogen, also anticipated the consequences of his discovery in his classical lectures on diabetes mellitus. Many investigators have made important observations in the sciences but only a few have recognized their ultimate significance. That is the greatness described by Schopenhauer: Many people find a stone but most throw it carelessly away without realizing its value; only a few keep it, polish it carefully until it is bright and shining, and reveal it to be a jewel.

All of his life von Pirquet was proud that he had discovered the significance of allergy. After World War I he was invited to lecture on this subject in the United States, where allergy had begun to develop into a special branch of medicine. Before leaving he let me read the manuscript. I called his attention to the latest American literature on the subject and advised him to quote a few of the authors. He smiled and said: "I don't think I will discuss the literature; I don't like it when someone else plays with my toy." There is deep truth in those simple words. For him research was not hard work but enjoyment, play, and gratification. He took the same pleasure from his other contributions to science, pediatrics, and medicine in general. The mental activities of children and of geniuses have features in common. Von Pirquet's character showed many childlike peculiarities. Schopenhauer said that every child is, as it were, a genius, and every genius is, so to speak, a child. The naïveté and exalted simplicity in von Pirquet's mentality were striking, and sometimes misunderstood.

Another peculiarity in von Pirquet's achievements which is found in the life history of other geniuses is the cyclical character of his productivity. Periods of intensive creativity alternated with periods when accomplishment ceased for lack of inspiration. In the former periods he shut himself away from others, concentrated on the problem he had in mind, and finished the work within a short time. In the latter periods he either played with his graphic hobbies or was idle and nonproductive and spent his time on nonessentials, waiting for new inspiration. Such periodic oscillation of creative power contrasts with the less variable life cycle of an average noncreative person.

Reading the scientific literature and the papers of others did not occupy much of his time. The scholar or teacher who is not a creative genius acquires his knowledge by thoroughly absorbing, digesting, and assimilating the work of others; the material is stored and can be produced if the need for it arises. By contrast, what did not come out of von Pirquet's own mind had little interest for him. The scholars among his contemporaries occasionally criticized his ignorance of the literature and even went so far as to say behind his back: "This man is finished." It did not occur to them that a genius might be measured by another yardstick. Geniuses should be judged by their highest achievements. To their work of inferior value Horace's words may be applied: *Quandoque bonus dormitat Homerus.*

Genius and erudition bear the same relation to one another as the text of an old classic to its commentary. All truth and all wisdom come first from direct observation and reasoning. Books do not replace experience; nor erudition, genius. Intrinsic wisdom is intuitive, not based on the ideas of others. A genius lives in a world apart. Natural intelligence can be extended to almost any degree by education, but education cannot replace natural intelligence. A single example from his own experience may teach a genius more than a scholar can learn from a thousand examples of others with which he had no personal encounter. Von Pirquet's lack of concern for what did not come from himself may have resulted because he felt that a continual influx of extraneous ideas would inhibit his own thoughts and that incessant reading and study would stultify the work of his brain.

In his research, three periods of creativity can be distinguished. The first was the bacteriological and immune-biological period from 1900 until 1913, culminating in the concept of allergy and the discovery of the tuberculin test. The second period, from 1914 until 1919, was devoted to anthropometrics and the science of nutrition. In the third period, during the 1920's, he occupied himself mainly with biometric and biostatistical studies. The individual periods are not sharply separated, but frequently overlap. His brilliant ideas on allergy and the tuberculin test were developed during his twenties and early thirties. During his forties, he devoted most of his time to his new system of nutrition. It was elaborated with the same vigor as his early achievements, but there were signs of intellectual decline and of peculiarities which revealed a slightly disturbed mind. The stronger term insanity is avoided.

Von Pirquet's studies on nutrition began during the second creative period. If it is correct to say that genius is assiduity, the aphorism would apply to that period, but assiduity as used here is more comparable with the *idée fixe* of a psychoneurotic. The assiduity is not extensive but intensive, directed toward a definite aim with single-minded passion. Four books and a dictionary of nutrition were the fruits of this period. His terminology was strange to the uninitiated and he had a strong tendency to replace description by formulae. The nutritional status of a child was expressed by a formula; vowels rather than digits were used for grading quantitative findings. He even tried to replace the form of routine case histories and records, which he considered long-winded and empty, by a condensed system of recording. He became almost fanatical on the subject. The interns had to pass an examination in the Pirquet system of nutrition; the nurses had to be trained to use it; and in the hospital the milk kitchen for infants and the diet kitchen for older children were operated according to his ideas. Special courses were arranged for the women who supervised the cooking and distribution of school lunches. The entire American Relief Administration was based on his nutritional system. Although the procedure encountered strong criticism, the basic idea of calculating nutritional requirements from the square of the sitting height rather than body weight was again the design of a genius.

Von Pirquet had an outstanding gift for mathematics and for graphic analysis of observations and phenomena. I can still see him in his shirt sleeves bending over a drawing board in his room at the *Kinderklinik*. He never worked at a desk but sat at a long table. He was fascinated by figures and seemed to prefer the slide rule to the stethoscope. Every chart, made with love and devotion, was a masterpiece. In later years his interest was concentrated more and more on vital statistics and biometrics. In 1927, he prepared a paper on the seasonal incidence of death, presented as a chart which resembled a map of the stars. When he was chairman of the League of Nations Committee for Child Hygiene, his main interest was vital statistics. After he had finished a paper and adorned it with drawings and charts, he would display it to his staff before it was read at a meeting. One might almost say that he liked to show it off, as an artist proudly displays his creations. Von Pirquet experienced the same elation from a chart he had constructed at the drawing board that another scientist derives from a successful experiment.

This taste for mathematics was exhibited not only in his own field. He liked to try out his artistic and constructional ideas in other realms as well. He built a special staircase at his house in the country that would conserve space; it was lost when the house was bombed. In one of his more playful moods he invented a card game of which he was very proud. Another invention was a gadget which would enable an automobile to be turned completely around on one spot. He registered the principle in the United States with the purpose of obtaining a patent, but it was buried in the "cemetery of inventions," his favorite term for the consignment of ephemeral ideas that never come to fruition.

All of this activity—the systematization, the device of a new language, and the inventions—is consistent with a schizothymic personality.

III

Married Life

While studying pediatrics in Berlin under Otto von Heubner, Clemens von Pirquet met a German girl one evening when he was attending the theater. Maria Christine van Husen of Hanover was twenty-two years old, four years his junior. She was employed in Berlin. They continued to see each other, and even after von Pirquet went to the *Kinderklinik* in Vienna he returned to Berlin to be with her whenever he could spare a weekend from his professional activities. A picture of Maria, taken when she was in the prime of her life, shows a woman of the type depicted by Rubens— buxom, with rosy cheeks and the appearance of one who enjoyed life.

A liaison such as this was not at all uncommon at the turn of the century for a young man of aristocratic family, but usually it was severed after a time and he chose a wife whose social background and interests were similar to his own. In 1904, however, Clemens and Maria Christine were married. This alliance was a bitter disappointment to the von Pirquet family, who took the position that Clemens had married beneath his station and made it clear to Maria that they did not accept her. Clemens' brother Silverio was the only member of the family who attended the wedding in Berlin, and he experienced a sense of foreboding that the marriage would be disastrous. Clemens' mother was heart-broken.

Little wonder that under those circumstances Maria Christine became more and more antagonistic and was at odds with everyone in her husband's family. One of Clemens' elder brothers mentioned an episode which he considered to have been an early factor in crystallizing the family attitude. A discussion had arisen as to what actions are or are not permitted in good society. Maria made the comment that anything not specifically forbidden was condoned provided one did not get caught. That rather harmless though slightly cynical remark, made in the presence of the children, was a red flag to a family whose conservative traditions

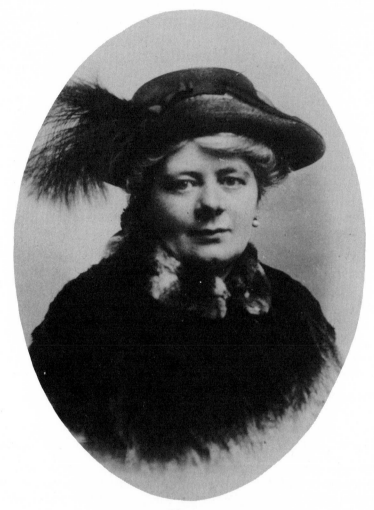

Maria Christine von Pirquet.

and early twentieth century moral standards were still unshaken. The ideas of her world and theirs clashed and she expressed her hostility quite openly. The constant bickerings and arguments made life difficult for Clemens, but he was devoted to his wife and remained faithful to her always. Friction in the family never ceased and more than a decade after the death of the mother, who divided the estate, it reached a point where the brothers and sisters brought lawsuits against Clemens and Maria over trifling differences concerning the distribution of the property in

Hirschstetten. The litigation was still unsettled at the time of their death.

Illness and an unsuccessful gynecological operation added to the trying situation. As a result of the surgery, Maria could never bear children. Many years later the couple adopted a son and a daughter. Although Clemens and Maria were fond of them and treated them kindly, the presence of their children did little to alleviate the tensions of an unhappy marriage.

Maria's physical state left its mark on body, soul, and mind. She aged early, became obese, spent most of the day in bed, smoked continually, and suffered from insomnia which necessitated the use of barbiturates. This medication led to a reversal of the normal cycle of night and day. During many a sleepless night she kept her husband awake reading to her—not always from good literature or writing which would have been of interest to him, but serialized fiction from the illustrated magazines. He would arrive at the hospital early on the morning after one of these episodes, so tired that he was apt to fall asleep whenever an opportunity arose. On such a morning one of his associates read to him a manuscript which he had written. Sitting in an easy chair, von Pirquet promptly dozed and waked only when the reading stopped. Without apology for not listening, he asked if there was not something more to be read so that he could continue the good sleep.

Maria made at least one attempt to commit suicide. She habitually took sleeping pills so that the opportunity for an overdose was always present. Because of her hysterical nature, however, the suicide attempt was thought to be only halfhearted, aimed chiefly at drawing attention to herself. Later she agreed to enter a private sanatorium near Vienna for treatment which it was hoped might wean her from her drug addiction. Her husband stayed with her at night and went daily to the *Kinderklinik*. She refused to co-operate and the experiment ended in failure after a few weeks.

In other moods she would be sociable, receive visitors, particularly foreigners of distinction, attend parties and, at certain festivals such as Christmas, visit the *Kinderklinik*. For a time she was caught up by the dancing mania of the postwar world.

When I met Maria first, in 1919, she was in bed. Although barely forty, she looked old, unkempt, and unattractive. Her speech was slurred from the effect of sleeping pills. Conversation was difficult and I had the feeling that von Pirquet would have preferred to cover up the unfavorable impression she made but at the same time he wanted to let me form my own opinion.

In only one instance that I can recall did she interfere at the *Kinderklinik*. That episode concerned a staff appointment. I was the personnel adviser and, having a free hand in appointing the interns and determining the duration of their tenure, I gave notice of termination to a woman physican at the end of her first year. She did not wish to relinquish her position, and realized her intention to stay by backstairs intrigue. Through the intervention of the "Frau Baronin" she was reinstated, and thereafter the two became intimate friends.

As so often happens, it is hard to distinguish between the somatic and the psychogenic components of Maria von Pirquet's ailments. Be that as it may, there is no essential difference between the two and it would be unjust to censure an unhappy woman afflicted with psychoneurosis. Her condition continued to deteriorate as the years passed.

The situation became especially difficult when she traveled with her husband to professional meetings. Most of the day she would remain in bed, but she liked to appear in the evening at social events. Frequently she could not avoid sleeping during the daytime, a situation which was particularly unfortunate when the von Pirquets had agreed to accept private hospitality.

All those who had insight into the married life of the couple knew how hard it was for von Pirquet. He could never be sure of what might happen and he never refused her demands. Frequently Maria would summon him home from the lecture room or from a meeting of the medical faculty. Unfortunately, her calls often came on the very occasions when it was most inconvenient for him to leave. When he had obligations or appointments outside the city, in which she could not be included, he would ask one of his friends to keep her company until his return. When she felt well he would occasionally telephone in the evening and invite me to his home for a game of bridge. One accepted for his sake; the game was not a pleasure because she had never mastered it. She had no real friends and no particular interests, although in her youth her contemporaries had regarded her as highly intelligent. When others were present she hid her dominating personality. She would call her husband *Clemchen* and be extremely kind and oversolicitous to him. A wife who appears too loving may torment her husband by her anxiety for his well-being, and satisfy her repressed hate by bursting into tears and making scenes until the unfortunate spouse is deprived of his personal liberty. Maria's jealousy was understandable if one takes into account that von Pirquet was still in the prime of life at a time when she was deteriorating rapidly.

The public was aware of the problem. It was impossible to conceal it. Gossip and idle criticism about the von Pirquets' married life flourished. The question was often asked why a man who was still youthful and attractive did not obtain a divorce and marry a more suitable partner; or why he did not at least let his wife be cared for in an institution so that he might lead a less disturbed private life which would permit greater concentration on his professional activities. Obviously in some way satisfaction outweighed dissatisfaction in his married life. A man is sometimes too proud to admit that he has made a mistake, but prefers to compromise and carry on somehow. Neither would it be consistent with von Pirquet's character to desert a sick woman. History records many cases in which a genius was reduced to a cipher at home by a wife who failed to understand him. Socrates and Xanthippe come to mind, and Goethe's marriage to Christiane Vulpius. Goethe fell in love with a girl of very humble station; he eventually married her, thereby causing endless scandal among the virtuous gossips of Weimar. A man who is less scrupulous and more determined, usually not a genius or a scholar, settles the problem more directly.

It would be easy to make Freudian interpretations of von Pirquet's marital problems, but only the obvious facts are presented here, the reader being left free to interpret them as he chooses. Of marriage in general von Pirquet once remarked: "It is a leap into darkness." It is not possible to analyze his deepest motives or why he never attempted to release himself from his bondage. The fact that he stayed with Maria to the end and arranged that she should share his grave of honor speaks for itself. It should be emphasized that in spite of his domestic problems he was able to pursue his professional goals until the last days of his life and to accomplish what he considered essential for completing the great scheme of productivity which he had started in his youth.

IV

Formative Years

After obtaining his degree in medicine, von Pirquet served six months as a medical officer in the armed forces and then went to Berlin for a short period of indoctrination in pediatrics under Otto von Heubner. By the end of 1901 he was ready to begin his training at the *Universitäts Kinderklinik* in Vienna, which at that time was housed in the St. Anna Children's Hospital. For two years he served as intern and resident under Theodor Escherich, and in 1903 he was advanced to the position of clinical assistant, the steppingstone to an academic career. Escherich's outstanding reputation had attracted a brilliant group of young physicians, including Franz Hamburger, who many years later succeeded von Pirquet as professor of pediatrics in Vienna; August Ritter von Reuss, noted for his studies of the newborn and author of the first textbook on the physiology and pathology of infants in that age group; Ludwig Jehle, known for his studies of orthostatic albuminuria; Bela Schick, von Pirquet's close friend and co-worker and the discoverer of the diphtheria test named for him; and Sluka and Egon Rach, who pioneered in pediatric radiology.

There existed a certain hierarchy based on seniority. The senior assistant's position was comparable to that of assistant to the physician-in-chief in the United States. He substituted for the chief in student lectures and examinations and carried out numerous administrative duties. He was, so to speak, the connecting link between the chief and the junior assistants. In general, relations among the assistants were smooth, although occasionally rivalry, jealousy, or friction developed as might be expected in any closely associated professional group, particularly if their respective areas of research overlap.

Such a disagreement arose between Hamburger and von Pirquet over the question of priority for the diagnostic tuberculin test. To be sure, Hamburger was correct in stating that von Pirquet was not the first to produce a tuberculin test. There had been precursors, an important one being Escherich's *Stichreaktion*

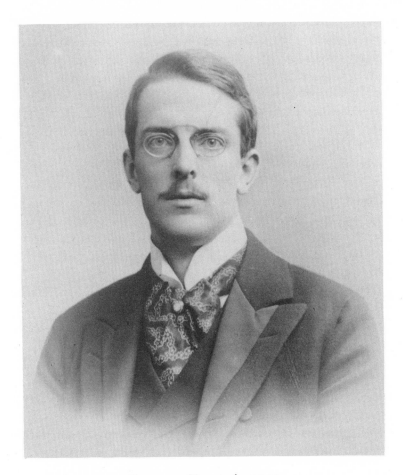

Clemens von Pirquet, about 1903.

(puncture test) which is characterized by swelling and redness following the subcutaneous injection of tuberculin. What made von Pirquet's test unlike the others was his simple, painless technique of applying the tuberculin to the surface of the slightly abraded skin. All of the other tuberculin tests of his day have long been abandoned, but the von Pirquet method is still in use. It was the first of his discoveries to reach beyond the medical profession and arouse the interest of the general public.

Von Pirquet's earliest paper, published in 1897 when he was a medical student at the University of Königsberg, is merely of historical interest. There were no trained laboratory technicians at that time and ambitious students were encouraged to participate in laboratory research at the university institutes. Although the student contributed few original ideas, he became familiar with research methods and with the scientific approach. Its limitations reminded him to be humble and modest and not to expect laboratory procedures to provide all the answers. (One of my friends suggested that Dante's advice to "abandon hope, all ye who enter here" should be written at the entrance to a research laboratory.) Von Pirquet's first paper, based on testing d'Arsonval's electrodes for uniformity and nonpolarizability, is a good example of this kind of student work. Contrary to d'Arsonval's theory, it indicated that the electrodes were by no means unpolarizable and could be considered uniform only under particularly favorable conditions. The head of the Department of Physiology, rather than von Pirquet, was primarily responsible for this polemic publication.[1]

In the second article of his formative years, published in 1902, von Pirquet entered the field of immunology in which he soon became famous. Although the problems were those generally discussed in the immunological literature of the period, they are of no particular interest and do not reflect his own ideas. The work was carried out in the university's Serotherapeutic Institute in collaboration with Rudolf Kraus, who was well known as the discoverer of specific precipitins in immune sera.[2]

Von Pirquet was particularly interested in studying the patient at bedside and in the third paper his own originality and independent thinking became evident. His investigation of the theory of serum sickness and incubation time was perceptive and detailed, and the preliminary report[3] gives evidence of the shape of things to come.

In a letter written from Munich he terminated an association with his first coworker on serum sickness, criticizing a lack of interest. The letter illustrates von Pirquet's straightforward attitude toward fundamental research, even at the risk of hurting the feelings of a friend.

---

[1] "Prüfung der d'Arsonval'schen Electroden auf Gleichartigkeit und Unpolarisirbarkeit," *Arch. f. d. ges. Physiol.* 65 (1897): 606.

[2] "Weitere Untersuchungen über spezifische Niederschläge," *Centralbl. f. Bakt.* 32 (1902): 60. (With R. Kraus.)

[3] "Sur la théorie de la période d'incubation," Congrès Internat. d'Hyg. et Démog., Brussels, Sept. 1903.

MUNICH, JUNE 24, 1903

DEAR FRIEND:

Many thanks for your letter of yesterday. It goes without saying that you will be mentioned in the paper. It was rather unpleasant for me to have to ask you to relinquish the work on serum sickness to Schick. However, you may have realized yourself that you were not making progress and were no longer interested, whereas Schick grasped the significance of the study, particularly its theoretical implications. He delved deeply into the problem with full vigor, at the expense of his spare time.

I am pleased that you wish to remain my coworker and I believe we may come to terms. By the way, I shall return to Vienna next week; we may talk about it some more.

Cordial greetings from your faithful friend Pirquet.

From then on Bela Schick collaborated in von Pirquet's research and became his loyal friend.

During his years as assistant at the *Kinderklinik*, von Pirquet devoted himself principally to his professional activities. His most masterly contributions to science appeared in rapid succession. Paul Moser, who introduced immune serum for scarlet fever, was first assistant of the clinic. Moser asked von Pirquet to collaborate in his studies on streptococci and the serum treatment of scarlet fever and it was he who discovered his young colleague's outstanding ability and guided him toward research. One publication on the agglutination of streptococci resulted from this collaboration.[4]

Streptococci from scarlet fever patients, cultured on artificial media for a considerable length of time, were agglutinated by an immune serum prepared by immunizing horses with the bacteria. The huge amounts of horse serum (up to 200 cc.) then used to treat patients provided von Pirquet with ample opportunity to observe the serum effect, and these observations soon crystallized into his theory of incubation time.

The study of incubation time by young von Pirquet was the turning point in his career and reveals his critical and scholarly mind in the most significant manner. Although still a coworker— this time of Max Gruber, professor of hygiene at the University of Munich, who had discovered that a causative organism was

[4] "Zur Agglutination der Streptokokken," *Centralbl. f. Bakt.* 34 (1903):560. (With P. Moser.)

agglutinated by the specific serum of patients suffering from the disease—von Pirquet's contribution was recognized as equal to that of the chief author. Gruber presented the study in 1903 to the Society of Morphology and Physiology in Munich, and published it with von Pirquet the same year. Entitled "Toxin and Antitoxin," it questions Ehrlich's side-chain theory.

An exchange of letters between the two authors throws light on von Pirquet's personality as well as his approach to the analysis of a scientific problem. Drafts of his own letters, as well as those from Gruber, were found among von Pirquet's literary legacy.[5] It is a sign of greatness rather than conceit to recognize early in life what should be preserved for posterity, and letters are among the most important documents.

Von Pirquet wrote first on June 2, 1903:

I have been informed by Prof. von Eiselsberg that you will be kind enough to listen to me.

My problem is dealing with observations on vaccination as well as with intensive studies of the morbid conditions almost invariably occurring in the human after administration of large doses of horse serum. I made these observations when a resident on the scarlet fever ward, where Moser's horse serum is administered in large doses.

Observations on the human as well as experimental investigations on animals have produced results which have great theoretical significance for the interpretation of infection, intoxication, and immunity. Since they are incompatible with Ehrlich's hypotheses and rather agree with your interpretation, I am getting in touch with you through Prof. v. Eiselsberg, and trust that you will be satisfied with my results.

Hoping to show you my material[6] soon in person I remain respectfully.

By return mail Gruber invited von Pirquet to Munich, although stating that he would be willing to discuss the problems by correspondence. Von Pirquet announced that he would arrive in Munich on June 10, believing that his investigations were so extensive that detailed discussion would be necessary in obtaining Gruber's opinion and advice. He continued:

As I remember, you mentioned once that a study of incubation time would furnish an important clue to the concept of immunity.

[5] The handwriting is sometimes difficult to decipher, particularly since several sentences were written in shorthand characters.

[6] The preceding April he had established priority by depositing at the Imperial Academy of Sciences in Vienna a short article, "On the Theory of Infectious Diseases."

The basic fact from which I start is that, in serum sickness as well as in vaccination, the time from the first intoxication or infection until occurrence of the specific reaction is rather constant, while the incubation time is always shorter after revaccination or reinjection. The detectable free antibodies show the same behavior. I shall pass on to you by word of mouth the conclusions drawn from these and other findings regarding the theory of immunity.

As von Pirquet indicated in his letters, Gruber's ideas did not coincide with those of Ehrlich. A brief summary will familiarize the reader with Ehrlich's theories about toxin and antitoxin.

Assuming that toxin and antitoxin would bind each other according to fixed stoichiometric relations and that the toxin-antitoxin complex was entirely nontoxic, Ehrlich expected that a mixture of the Lo-dose[7] of toxin with one-tenth of the immunizing unit of antitoxin would lose one-tenth of its toxicity. In other words, he believed that a toxin solution which contained 100 lethal doses per unit of volume would retain 90 lethal doses after admixture with one-tenth of the amount of antiserum necessary for complete neutralization. The experimental findings, however, disclosed that the mixture in which only a tenth part of the affinity of the toxin to the antitoxin was saturated produced only 70 per cent or less of the full toxic effect. The addition of three-tenths of the neutralizing amount of antiserum sometimes destroyed 80 or 85 per cent of the toxicity, while an additional seven-tenths had to be added in order to eliminate this 15 or 20 per cent of toxicity. Ehrlich concluded that the affinity to antitoxin should be sharply distinguished from the toxic effect itself; the former he attributed to a "haptophore," the latter to a "toxophore" atom complex.

The conclusion from Ehrlich's experiments on fractional neutralization and from his concept of a separate affinity and toxicity is that the toxins in solution differ in their degree of toxicity and their avidity for the antitoxin. Ehrlich supposed that the bacterial toxins also contained weakly toxic substances, the toxones, having slight avidity for antitoxin. Since the addition of one-tenth or more of an antitoxin solution did not produce decreased toxicity, Ehrlich further assumed that sometimes "toxoids" were also present which had the same number of haptophore groups as the toxins, but no toxophore groups. Depending upon the degree of their avidity for antitoxins in comparison with the avidity of the

---

[7] Amount of a toxin solution which can be added to the immunizing unit of an antitoxin solution without causing any toxic effects; it is the maximum amount of toxin which can be just neutralized by a given amount of antitoxin.

toxins, Ehrlich distinguished such forms as protoxoids, syntoxoids, and epitoxoids. He presented the result of his fractional titration by the so-called toxin spectrum: The abscissa was divided into equal sections corresponding to the number of haptophore groups; the length of the Y-axis was proportional to the number of toxophore groups. The different toxins, toxoids, and toxones followed from left to right according to their avidity for antitoxin, that is, in the order in which they were neutralized by fractional admixture of antitoxin.

In a lecture delivered in Vienna in 1901, Gruber had stated that Ehrlich's conclusions on neutralization were untenable and that it was a misconception for Ehrlich to believe he could carry out chemical analyses by physiological methods. He questioned that free toxin would act in the same manner under all circumstances or that conclusions about the binding of toxins could be drawn from the absence or change of the toxin effect, which might be inhibited or furthered by various foreign substances and under various conditions.

Gruber cited an experiment of Dreyer and Madsen, who at that time still firmly supported Ehrlich. They had observed that a mixture of a certain diphtheria toxin with antitoxin, given to a guinea pig, no longer contained free toxin but had 33 free toxon equivalents. However, in the rabbit the same mixture exerted marked toxin effect and contained 33 free toxin equivalents in addition to 40 free toxon equivalents. This one experiment proved decisively to Gruber the ineffectiveness of Ehrlich's toxin analysis and his lack of insight into chemistry. (Ehrlich maintained that he could titrate off one toxin after the other.) Unfortunately Gruber was unable to provide a comprehensive theory to replace Ehrlich's. Von Pirquet's graphic analysis and mathematical ingenuity explained the action of an antitoxin on a toxin and provided Gruber with a welcome stimulus for carrying out experiments to invalidate Ehrlich's theories.

Gruber was so impressed by von Pirquet's findings that he wrote to him a few days after their meeting in Munich:

You made a point-blank shot with your calculation of Madsen's experiments. I have carried out some experiments during the last three days with a known toxin, the uniformity of which cannot be in doubt. I succeeded in demonstrating a successive weakening of the action of toxin by addition of antitoxin (charts included).[8] Just for fun I include also Ehrlich's toxin spectrum.

These experiments have clarified with one stroke the most obscure details in the history of a toxin, e.g., the "toxoid formation."

I am of the opinion that you should not hesitate to publish your charts. Before September somebody else may take the same approach. You may have talked about it?

I should like to suggest the *Münchener medizinische Wochenschrift* and would publish my experiments in connection with your notice. If you prefer, I would also be willing to publish in collaboration with you; it goes without saying that priority for the calculations would be attributed to you alone.

With best congratulations and greetings.

Another enthusiastic letter from Gruber followed the next day:

I performed a new experiment today by a still more refined technique which shows the ridiculousness of Ehrlich's toxin theory, on the one hand, and the mode of reaction of antitoxins, on the other. The new theory is ready and sheds additional light on the problem in a surprising manner. One important point is now open to an experimental approach. Would you not like to study the problem together with me? I should like to show my thanks to you for letting me in on the secret of your work and for giving me the incentive for more thorough consideration. If you are dispensable in Vienna, leave everything behind and come straight away to Munich. . . .

The success of the experiments which I have in mind is certainly dubious. They may prove negative; however, this does not mean that the theory is wrong as the experimental conditions are highly involved. If they prove positive the triumph is still greater. Your ideas on the relations of toxin to antitoxin are only partly correct. We experiment also in this direction. The experiments have to be carried out even more exactly.

Please think it over.

One day later Gruber hastily sent a postcard to von Pirquet:

I am sorry to tell you the proposed experiments are unnecessary, since Madsen himself has already calculated and drawn the chart which you recently presented to me. He reached all the conclusions from his study. I discovered it yesterday in the *Festskrift ved indvielsen* of Statens Serum Institute (1902) and shall now publish the confirming experiments.

[8] Of the total amount of toxin, 95.5% is made ineffective by the first 3/10 of antitoxin; for the last 4.5%, 6/10 are required. In a second experiment, 92.1% of toxin was destroyed by the first 2/7 or 3/10 of antitoxin.

Von Pirquet answered by return mail:

I was very pleased that you were able to confirm immediately my calculations of the toxin-antitoxin effect by experiment and to find such satisfactory agreement. In your second experiment it is striking that the decrease of the toxin effect is relatively small following addition of 1/10 antitoxin. This irregularity of the curve is not present in Madsen's experiment, but an intimation can be noticed in Ehrlich's experiment which I analyzed. Anyway, Ehrlich must have observed this phenomenon several times; otherwise he would not have invented the less toxic prototoxoid. According to our assumption the other toxoids or toxons are nothing but attenuated full toxin; it is irrelevant whether the attenuation resulted from addition of antitoxin or from other procedures, such as effect of light, electricity, oxygen, etc.[9] . . .

For the remaining part of the curves, my conclusions from the analysis of Madsen's experiments are valid in any case:

1. The attenuation of a toxin by addition of antitoxin does not take place in linear proportion or by leaps (Ehrlich) but according to a curve of higher order.

2. A toxin attenuated by heat behaves like one attenuated by addition of an antitoxin.

3. Ehrlich's assumption that the binding (haptophore) capability is unchangeable is incorrect and due to an error of observation.

4. Therefore, we have no reason to assume a difference of individual toxin groups within the toxins heretofore studied (tetanolysin, agglutinins, staphylolysin, ricin).

I think that publication of the results is not urgent. I should like to wait, if possible, until September. I have talked only with a few intimate friends here about the theories (with my coworker Schick, and also with Drs. Moser, Hamburger, and Sperk).

In his reply Gruber re-emphasized the urgency of immediate publication:

. . . for Ehrlich knows already through Madsen that his theory is untenable and will probably himself present his altered views at the Congress in Brussels. In addition, Madsen has obviously not yet drawn conclusions from his studies because of his regard for Ehrlich. They go much further than you yourself surmise, as I realize from your letter. Excuse me for not detailing them to you, but I have had bad experiences about the unbelievable rapidity with which such things seep through.

---

[9] Similar opinions were held by Bordet (*Ann. de l'Instit. Pasteur* [1903], p. 161), and von Behring. A toxin becomes attenuated from attacking all sorts of chemical radicals.

Let us publish the experiments together. You have given me the incentive, but on the other hand you have not had enough chemical training to draw all the conclusions yourself. These conclusions, however, are of enormous significance.

Is it immodest that I ask you to come to Munich once more? We can then discuss everything thoroughly, go over the literature and write the article together. . . .

Von Pirquet's files contained no copy of his response, but the article with Gruber was published soon thereafter.

When Gruber first presented the data at Munich he stated: "Sometime ago, Herr Dr. Cl. Freiherr v. Pirquet came to see me. In addition to other interesting experimental results and considerations of his studies with Dr. B. Schick, he presented to me a chart obtained from calculating Madsen's experimental results on the neutralization of tetanolysin by its antitoxins."[10] (Fig. 1.)

Instead of calculating the percentage of toxic effect removed by each aliquot of the neutralizing amount of antitoxin, von Pirquet's chart recorded the fractions of toxic effect remaining after addition of the antitoxin portions. To understand the curve, it must be remembered that in the culture media of the tetanus bacillus, tetanolysin, which has the peculiarity of hemolyzing red blood cells, is formed in addition to the tetanus antitoxin. This capability is quantitatively limited in that only a precise maximum of red blood cells can be hemolyzed by a certain quantity of tetanus toxin solution. A fixed volume of antitoxin solution is necessary if hemolysis is to be completely prevented within a precise period of time (point of neutralization). When only fractions of this completely neutralizing antiserum are added to the toxin solution, hemolysis is more or less limited. One can determine from the amount of hemolyzed hemoglobin exactly which fraction of the total toxin solution has remained after addition of the serum.

The curve showed that the neutralization process proceeded at a steady rate, unlike the zigzag of Ehrlich's toxin spectrum. In view of von Pirquet's chart, Gruber felt everyone would agree that the postulation of diverse toxins in tetanolysin was entirely untenable. Moreover, the chart explained the mysterious antitoxin effect.

[10] Thorvald Madsen, "Ueber Tetanolysin," *Ztschr. f. Hyg. u. Infektionskr.* 32: 225.

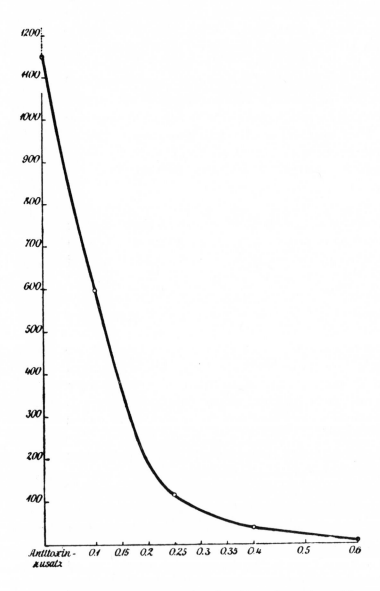

Fig. 1. Von Pirquet's curve prepared from Madsen's experimental data. (Vertical scale—Effect of toxin; Horizontal scale—Addition of antitoxin.) *From:* Gruber, M. and v. Pirquet, C. "Toxin und Antitoxin," *München. med. Wchnschr.* 50: (1903): 1193. (Courtesy of J. F. Lehmanns Verlag, Munich.)

If toxin and antitoxin interacted like a strong acid and a strong alkali, which Ehrlich had assumed to be self-evident, each aliquot of antitoxin would bind an equivalent share of toxin and destroy an equivalent fraction of the toxic effect. In that event the line combining the terminal points of the *Y*-axis, indicating what percentage of toxic effect remained, would be a straight line reaching the abscissa at the point of neutralization. An asymptotic curve represents a reaction between two compounds with weak affinity which never arrive at complete neutralization. The tetanolysin curve is of the same character as the so-called reversible reactions of dissociable compounds, or the reactions of electrolytes, or those of molecular compounds in varying proportions with decreasing affinity.

Electrolytic dissociation in the narrower sense of ionization of the compound toxin-antitoxin and hydrolysis—as, for instance, the splitting of stannic chloride by water into hydrochloric acid and stannic hydrate—can be ruled out since toxin and antitoxin are nonelectrolytic organic compounds. There is only a question of the usual dissociation, such as that of the salts of weak alkalis and acids or of molecular compounds in varying proportions.

Gruber and von Pirquet described a chemical reaction analogous to the interaction of toxin and antitoxin, such as the heat production of sulfuric acid hydrate and water. The first molecule of water added to pure sulfuric acid hydrate produces approximately 6,300 calories of heat, the second only 3,000 calories, and so on with rapid decrease; but even the 1,600th water molecule causes positive heat production. The magnitude of heat production is the index of the affinity between varying concentrations of sulfuric acid and water.

Figures 2 and 3 present further analogies to the toxin-antitoxin interaction. Because of its extreme affinity for water, concentrated sulfuric acid decomposes cane sugar the same as other organic substances under carbonization, but this is not true of dilute sulfuric acid. Sulfuric acid is therefore a toxin for cane sugar, water an antitoxin of sulfuric acid for cane sugar (Fig. 2). After the steep drop at the outset a long trail with minimal gradient follows, just as the first tenth of tetanus antitoxin eliminates a disproportionate fraction of the toxicity of tetanus toxin while the last vestiges of toxicity are difficult to eradicate.

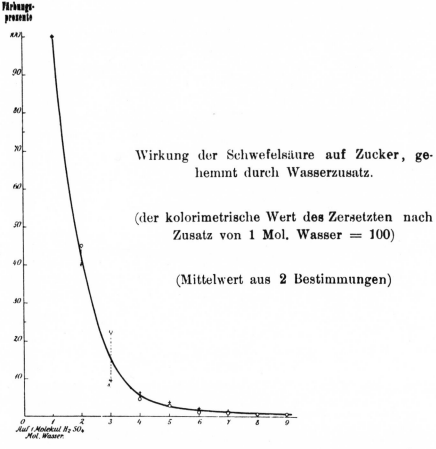

Färbungs-
prozente

Wirkung der Schwefelsäure **auf Zucker**, ge-
hemmt durch Wasserzusatz.

(der kolorimetrische Wert des Zersetzten nach
Zusatz von 1 Mol. Wasser = 100)

(Mittelwert aus 2 Bestimmungen)

Auf 1 Molekul $H_2 SO_4$
Mol. Wasser.

Fig. 2. Effect of sulfuric acid on sugar, inhibited by addition of water. Colorimetric value of disintegrated material after addition of 1 mol. water = 100. (Mean value from two determinations.) (Vertical scale—% of staining; Horizontal scale—Mol. water per 1 mol. H_2SO_4.) *From:* Gruber, M. and v. Pirquet, C. "Toxin und Antitoxin," *München. med. Wchnschr.* 50 (1903): 1193. (Courtesy of J. F. Lehmanns Verlag, Munich.)

Figure 3 presents another example of molecular compounds with decreasing affinity. The strong osmotic pressure of water on the red blood cells causes them to swell and leads to the escape of hemoglobin. However, water containing a sufficient amount of sodium chloride produces no effect on the red blood cells. Water is therefore a toxin for the erythrocytes, sodium chloride its anti-toxin. The addition of graduated amounts of sodium chloride gradually abolishes the toxicity of water by successively diminishing the affinity and thereby the osmotic pressure. Figure 4 shows "a toxin spectrum of water" according to Ehrlich's interpretation,

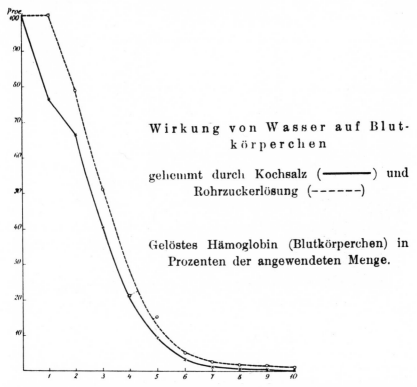

Fig. 3. Effect of water on red blood cells inhibited by sodium chloride (solid line) and cane sugar solution (broken line). Dissolved hemoglobin (red blood cells) in per cent o the amount used. (Vertical scale—%; Horizontal scale—Units of antitoxin.) *From:* Gruber, M. and v. Pirquet, C. "Toxin und Antitoxin," *München. med. Wchnschr.* 50 (1903): 1193. (Courtesy of J. F. Lehmanns Verlag, Munich.)

with proto-, deutero-, tritotoxins, toxons, and even a protoxoid. Depending upon which antitoxin is used, an entirely different series of toxins, i.e., different relations of the toxophore to the haptophore groups, can be found in the same water.

Arrhenius, who discovered electrolytic dissociation, and Madsen, an outstanding pupil of Ehrlich, settled the question. They ascertained that the toxin-antitoxin neutralization curve proceeds within certain limits in the same manner as the curve of neutralization of ammonia by boric acid. In both processes the actual state of equilibrium between the unbound and bound shares of the two substances is expressed by the formula:

$$\left\{\frac{\text{Free toxin}}{\text{Volume}}\right\} \left\{\frac{\text{Free antitoxin}}{\text{Volume}}\right\} = K \left\{\frac{\text{Compound toxin-antitoxin}}{\text{Volume}}\right\} 2$$

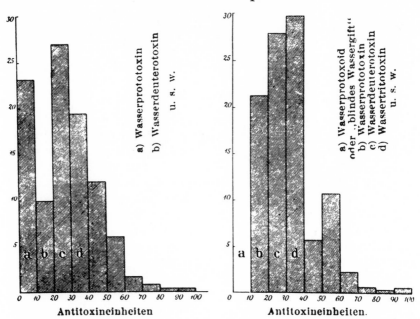

Fig. 4. Toxin spectrum of water with sodium chloride (left) and cane sugar (right). Left: *a* = water prototoxin; *b* = water deuterotoxin, etc. Right: *a* = water protoxoid or "blind water toxin"; *c* = water deuterotoxin; *d* = water tritotoxin, etc. (Vertical scales—% of toxophore groups; Horizontal scales—Antitoxin units.) *From*: Gruber, M. and v. Pirquet, C. "Toxin und Antitoxin," *München. med. Wchnschr.* 50 (1903): 1193. (Courtesy of J. F. Lehmanns Verlag, Munich.)

Only the constant, K, of the two processes is different. One molecule of toxin and one of antitoxin form one molecule compound, a reaction which is never quite completed. The observed and the calculated values agree so exactly that no doubt about the nature of the tetanolysin process can remain. Arrhenius and Madsen had obviously concluded that Ehrlich's theory was buried, but they did not draw all the conclusions which were possible.[11]

After the article was published Ehrlich sent a reply to the same journal; his remarks were just as acrid as Gruber and Pirquet's. He defended his side-chain theory, clung to the concept of the plurality of toxins, and disputed the validity of Gruber's experiments. The journal editor sent galley proofs to Gruber, who forwarded them to von Pirquet with the comments: "I can't accept the toxoid formation, at least not yet; Ehrlich can start his system

[11] "Toxin und Antitoxin," *München. med. Wchnschr.* 50 (1903): 1193, 1259. (With M. Gruber.)

all over again. I don't find that Ehrlich produces very fundamental material, just new hypotheses again and again. Why he
provided entirely different toxin spectra of water, I am unable to
explain at present."

Von Pirquet's answer was somewhat critical:

The difference between your toxin spectrum of water and Ehrlich's
can be explained in the following manner: You ascertained in your preliminary experiment the zone in which in general an attenuation of the
water effect by cane sugar took place, and divided this zone, *AB*, into
10 parts. However, there is no statement about this preliminary experiment in either *Wiener klinische Wochenschrift* or *Münchener medizinische Wochenschrift*. . . . It must be admitted that Ehrlich's objection
is justified in view of our inexact record of the experiment, but Ehrlich
shirked the essential like a lawyer. His arguments for the toxoid formation (one experiment by himself, one by Madsen, and the statement of
Arrhenius and Madsen on diphtheria—not tetanus toxin examined by
Madsen in 1899) are sparse, but counter-evidence is not at all in our
interest.

Ehrlich's experiment contradicting Danysz[12] proves only that after
15 minutes an almost definite binding between toxin and antitoxin has
taken place. Differences in the velocity of reaction can still result if
injection is made within a shorter interval. Thus it is not proved that
the diphtheria toxin and its antitoxin behave like strong acids and
bases. One can declare with certainty that the diphtheria antitoxin in
principle would not be different from the tetanus antitoxin. That
Ehrlich does not go to the heart of the matter, and considers the work
of Arrhenius and Madsen only a disclosure of an immaterial source of
error, really gave me much pleasure. In this way he puts himself in a
bad light. . . . Of great importance seems to me Madsen and Dreyer's
proof of the toxin effect of a tenfold amount of a mixture which contains only toxons. It is unwise of Ehrlich to mention this argument
spontaneously, since his explanation of the residual amounts of toxin is
defensible only if he assumes a compound with weak affinity. He limits
the spectrum considerably and therefore admits the inaccuracy of his
fundamental method. Ehrlich again follows the tactics which you previously characterized at the Medical Society in Vienna: he assails the
weak stand to distract attention from the position to which he has to
retreat. He does not look into the principal matter at all, namely, that
the saturation curve in the case of tetanolysin represents an asymptotic

[12] This refers to a statement by Danysz that the power of neutralization
changes on standing over a longer period of time. Danysz attributed the change
to an altered velocity of reaction.

curve and is compatible with the reaction of two compounds with weak affinity. Finally, it is nonessential whether or not the comparative curves are correctly applied. You have explicitly contrasted the molecular and the dissociable compounds.

We have for several reasons given considerable space to this work and to the exchange of letters between the noted professor and world-renowned scholar and the young, unknown resident of the *Kinderklinik*. It was von Pirquet's first great achievement in the science of immunology, and he reached his conclusions through graphic analysis and construction. A curve did not serve simply to illustrate text, it was a scientific technique which led to success in his later research. Ehrlich was at that time the outstanding expert in the field of immune biology. His side-chain theory, although only an auxiliary hypothesis in the interpretation of toxin and antitoxin effect on an organism, without experimental proof, was as generally accepted as the revelation on Mount Sinai. To question or criticize it was almost heresy.

In their collaboration, Gruber provided the driving aggressive force, possibly because of ambition and jealousy.[13] Von Pirquet's work on incubation time and serum sickness together with his analysis and calculation of Madsen's curve provided Gruber with a welcome opportunity for attacking Ehrlich. Gruber's letters clearly illustrate his attitude. Heated discussions, sometimes even with personal invective, were not uncommon in the German scientific literature. They sprang from the same spirit which gave rise to the dueling students' fraternities. This kind of polemic in the field of science does not often exist in the Anglo-Saxon countries. Freedom of speech provides sufficient outlet for aggression in the democracies. Von Pirquet himself was rarely a fighter unless his own theories were attacked.

Von Pirquet first publicly discussed vaccination in connection with his fundamental antigen-antibody theory in 1903, before the pediatric section of the Society of German Natural Scientists and Physicians, in Cassel. He stated that since the specific reaction due to vaccination is not produced by the invading virus, it must be conditioned by the other pertinent factor, namely, the invaded organism. The body does not act as a passive culture medium; the onset of disease may be considered a positive reaction of the organism toward the intruder. The antibodies which produce

[13] He was a fanatic teetotaler. Aggressiveness is occasionally characteristic.

this reaction develop several days after the first vaccination and in a much shorter time after subsequent vaccination. He emphasized the analogy to serum sickness and denied the validity of Ehrlich's side-chain theory in immune biology.[14]

In 1904 von Pirquet read a paper before the Society of German Natural Scientists and Physicians, in Breslau, on determinations of body weight in acute nephritis. In the course of the disease, increased weight due to water retention usually precedes the occurrence of albuminuria. Weight loss, on the other hand, ushers in the convalescent period even while albuminuria still persists.[15] Although this observation has little diagnostic importance today, it fit well into von Pirquet's ideas at that time. Edema is one of the signs of serum sickness, and he was quick to recognize the nephritis following scarlet fever as an antigen-antibody reaction. Later he called it "eczema of the kidney." After he evolved the concept of serum sickness, he had almost a compulsion to apply its basic mechanism whenever it could be justified.

Another paper of von Pirquet's early period, published with Schick on the theory of "aggressin," shows how the new concept of serum sickness replaced shaky auxiliary hypotheses by a sound, simple theory. The term "aggressin" had been coined by Bail, an immunologist. He explained the sudden death of tubercular guinea pigs following reinjection with tubercle bacilli, or the death of normal animals after they had been injected with peritoneal exudates and bacilli recovered from tubercular guinea pigs, as resulting from the aggressive effect of the bacteria. He considered aggressin to be a mysterious immunological compound which paralyzed the leukocytes that were the animal's defense mechanism. Instead of this rather artificial theory, von Pirquet and Schick's interpretation was that the hypersensitivity of tubercular guinea pigs and the effect of peritoneal exudates were conditioned by antibody-like reaction products of the infected organism.[16]

Von Pirquet's gift for introducing technical innovations sometimes extended beyond his own field. Two of his publications were

[14] *Zur Theorie der Vaccination, Verhandlungen der 20. Versammlung der Gesellschaft fur Kinderheilkunde* . . . (Wiesbaden: J. F. Bergmann, 1904), p. 156.

[15] *Körpergewichtsbestimmungen bei Nephritis, Verhandlungen der 21. Versammlung der Gesellschaft fur Kinderheilkunde* . . . (Wiesbaden: J. F. Bergmann, 1905), p. 1.

[16] "Zur Frage des Aggressins," *Wien. klin. Wchnschr.* 18 (1905): 531. (With B. Schick.)

of this order. One dealt with an apparatus for the sterile injection of fluid in quantities of 1,000 cc. or more, particularly scarlet fever serum or physiological saline. His principle was to replace an ordinary plunger-type syringe by a simple air pump, thus distributing the necessary force by multiple ejections of the air column in the pump. Because the air does not come into direct contact with the fluid to be injected, the pump need not be sterilized.[17] The other publication described a windowed tongue depressor consisting of a piece of nickel wire with fused ends and prongs like those of a pair of pliers. The window permitted inspection of the buccal mucosa, particularly for Koplik's spots.[18]

In 1906, while writing a monograph on vaccinial immunity, von Pirquet became aware of the inadequacy of the word "immunity" to represent the manifold effects on the body of a first vaccination and revaccinations. His monograph, "Clinical Studies on Vaccination and Vaccinial Allergy," was published the next year.[19] For this fundamental work he was given the advanced academic title of *Privatdozent* (university lecturer) of pediatrics by the University of Vienna. In an illuminating article, Hans Schadewaldt credits pediatrics with having produced the theory of allergy.[20] Both the early reaction in revaccination and the positive tuberculin test are allergic manifestations. Later the term allergy acquired a broader meaning and now has been applied to a special branch of medicine.

As early as 1875, Bohn stated in his textbook of vaccination: "Being accessible to experimentation as hardly any other field of pathology, the theory of vaccination should develop into an exact chapter of pathology." He complained that the literature on smallpox vaccination had gained more in width than in depth. In the introduction to his monograph von Pirquet mentioned that the most modern textbook of his time, Krehl's *Pathological Physiology*, contained no mention of vaccination. His own penetrating clinical observations filled this gap 107 years after Jenner's

[17] "Apparat zur sterilen Injektion grösserer Flüssigkeitsmengen, speziell Scharlach-Serum und steriler Kochsalzlösung" (Vienna: G. Moser, 1904).

[18] "Gefensterter Mundspatel aus Nickeldraht," *München. med. Wchnschr.* 51 (1904): 1693.

[19] *Klinische Studien über Vaccination und vaccinale Allergie* (Vienna: Franz Deuticke, 1907). (Courtesy of Franz Deuticke, Vienna.)

[20] Hans Schadewaldt, "Die geschichtliche Bedeutung der Pädiatrie für die Entwicklung der Allergie," *Medizinische* 14 (1959): 681.

discovery. Von Pirquet's previous studies on serum sickness, incubation time, hypersensitiveness, and accelerated reaction furnished the solid foundation for this exhaustive monograph on vaccination. It is so complete that we may say without exaggeration that no essential progress has been made since that time (Figs. 5–7).

Von Pirquet's investigations started with a study of the progressive course of the phenomena of disease. He interpreted the *Frühreaktion* (early reaction) as an immediate allergic response, differing from that of a first vaccination. Up to that time the medical profession rarely repeated a vaccination because it was believed that an initial inoculation produced lasting immunity. Von Pirquet made many of his observations from repeated vaccinations on his own arm. Earlier he had observed at the bedside that the manifestations after a first injection of horse serum did not occur for at least ten days; after a second injection, the interval was shorter and the effect was sometimes observed even in the course of the same day. He found the most striking analogy to this phenomenon in vaccination, where the difference between immediate and accelerated reaction was also recognized.

After repeated smallpox inoculations, the occurrence of symptoms is related to the interval which has elapsed since the initial vaccination. First is a period of complete insensitivity; second,

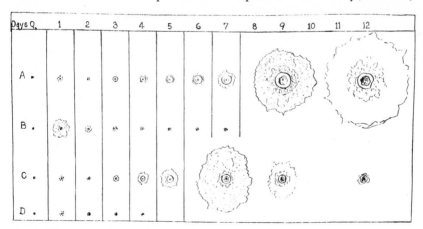

Fig. 5. Daily observation of cowpox vaccination in man. *A*. First vaccination with cowpox. *B*. Revaccination after short interval; early reaction. *C*. Revaccination after long interval. *D*. Trauma only. *From:* "Allergy," *Arch. Int. Med.* 7 (1911): 383. (Courtesy of American Medical Association, Chicago.)

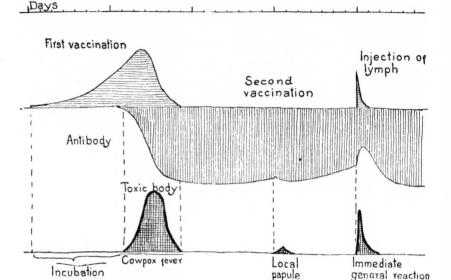

Fig. 6. Effects of first and repeated cowpox vaccination in man. *From:* "Allergy," *Arch.
Int. Med.* 7 (1911): 383. (Courtesy of American Medical Association, Chicago.)

an immediate reaction; and third, an accelerated ability to react.
If revaccination follows within a few weeks of the primary vaccination, the concentration of antibodies circulating in the blood
is so high that the few vaccinial organisms entering the body are
immediately destroyed (complete insensitivity). If approximately
two years have elapsed, a slight redness usually appears at the
site of vaccination within twenty-four hours, occasionally with a
small vesicle in the center. This represents an immediate ability
to react, or an immune reaction. According to von Pirquet's
theory, the concentration of antibodies has already decreased in
this instance. Although they suffice to kill the vaccinial organism,
they are no longer sufficient to digest immediately the toxic
products of disintegration. The result is an inflammatory reaction
at the site of the revaccination without scar formation. If the
period of time between primary vaccination and revaccination
is four to five years or more, the reaction takes place even earlier.
On the fourth or fifth day a small vesicle develops, which quickly
dries up and leaves a fine scar. We may suppose that in this instance the specific antibodies are almost entirely missing, but
they can be produced much faster than in the unvaccinated in-

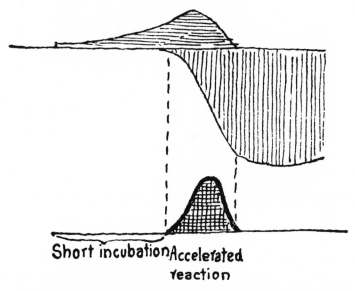

Fig. 7. Second cowpox vaccination after long interval. *From:* "Allergy," *Arch. Int. Med.* 7 (1911): 383. (Courtesy of American Medical Association, Chicago.)

dividual and can attack the vaccinial organism before they are fully developed (accelerated reaction).

His treatise on vaccination established both a theory of immunity and a concept of the origin of manifestations of disease. Previously these manifestations had been considered simply a result of the absorption of bacteria or their toxins. Fever was believed to be a sign of the systemic invasion of the organism; incubation time, either the period during which reproduction of the causative organism reached a threshold beyond which it became a menace to the body or the interval necessary to form a new generation of the causative organism. Von Pirquet considered the *onset* of signs of illness, not their *termination*, a symptom of antibody formation.

He drew a curve to depict the local symptoms of first vaccination, since daily millimetric measurements were required to establish an exact basis for comparison with revaccination. By recognizing the essential difference between development of the papilla, on the one hand, and the areola and *Frühreaktion*, on the other, he modified his original hypothesis that antibodies were responsible for the entire vaccinial reaction: "I now can distinguish manifestations predominantly depending upon the development of the infectious agent from those predominantly attributable to the effect of antibodies."

These ideas were expressed for the first time in his monograph. He also clarified the understanding of varioloid, which he interpreted as a typical reaction to the smallpox virus in those individuals who had either been vaccinated a long time before or had recovered from smallpox. Varioloid, like revaccination after a long interval, is an allergic modification of the variola process.

As the discoverer of an important new concept in a field not his own, von Pirquet had to defend the existence of a vaccinial early reaction of the "immune" organism against an expert in this field, the immunologist Kraus, with whom he had once collaborated. At a meeting of the medical society in Vienna on February 22, 1907, von Pirquet read a paper describing his theory of the skin rash in smallpox. He explained the symptoms following vaccinial early reaction, first vaccination, and smallpox by inoculation (variola inoculata). The antibodies leading to eruption of the skin rash might be agglutinins; by their activity the smallpox organisms circulating in the blood stream form clumps which cannot pass through the capillaries. They still contain viable organisms which grow into new colonies at sites where conditions for their further development are favorable—i.e., in the epithelium—while they perish inside the body.

In the subsequent discussion, Kraus bitingly attacked both von Pirquet's agglutination theory and his explanation of the early reaction in revaccination. The next discussor, Escherich, was more conciliatory: "Kraus's critical remarks cannot spoil my enjoyment in the keen ideas of the speaker." He agreed that not all of the hypotheses were convincing and felt that the weakest point was the theory of the variola exanthema. However, he considered the nucleus of von Pirquet's presentation to be his theory that the onset of illness is elicited by the occurrence of antibodies, a surprising concept obviously related to earlier work on serum sickness. Escherich considered the concept of incubation time to be not a simple statement of fact but a true biological law. Vaccinations repeated on successive days provided convincing proof that the local reaction was not stimulated by the amount of infectious organisms or the development of a local focus but by a general cause omnipresent in the entire organism.

Von Pirquet's concluding remarks are translated verbatim:

Professor Kraus in essence denies any scientific justification whatsoever of my theory. In fact, I am happy about this vigorous disagreement, since it proves the great difference between my interpretation and that accepted hitherto. It protects me against the danger of having somebody say later, when my ideas have prevailed: We have known that for a long time.

If Kraus denies me the right to express my opinion on the origin of an exanthema because each has its unexplained peculiarities, he thereby rejects the justification of any theory. I did not present my deliberations as facts, but emphatically emphasized their hypothetical character.

Regarding the facts, Kraus had to admit that the "early reaction" in serum sickness and vaccination indeed exists, which he previously questioned. As to the transmission of the early reaction, he obviously misunderstood me last year: I expected that the vesicle of my early reaction would not be transmissible; this was indeed the case. It is a fact that the small vaccinial reactions are not transmissible. This is well known to all inoculators and was proven a hundredfold by animal vaccination. I found interesting proof in the literature. One of the inoculators a hundred years ago used to test smallpox vaccine on his hand. If a papule developed there, the material was considered effective for use.

Kraus is in error when he states that antibodies have not been identified in the variola-vaccinial process. The studies of Beclère, Chambon, and Ménard, carried out with great exactness, show that an antivirulent, probably bactericidal, substance appears in the serum of vaccinated individuals at the same time the virulence of the pustular content dies out. The appearance of bacteriolytic antibodies, which I postulate, occurs a few days earlier; I explain the difference by quantitative conditions of saturation.

On the strength of the early reaction in serum sickness and vaccination, I affirm that we are justified in applying to antibody reactions conclusions drawn from vital processes. We have here just as specific reactions as the antibody reactions hitherto observed *in vitro*. Although the pathologists have guided us in this direction—and Kraus as an immunologist and the discoverer of precipitin reactions stands in the forefront—they are not yet willing to take this step from the theoretical to the practical. I am convinced that clinical elaboration will uphold the antibody theory.[21]

As a matter of fact his theory was upheld, although the discussion on antibodies which von Pirquet had in mind in his concept of infectious allergy still continues. In a short article he clarified his point of view and separated *immunity* from what he thereafter called *allergy*.[22] The question remains whether immunity and hypersensitivity are linked or whether the process causing immunity by prior treatment is separate from that leading to hypersensitivity. Wolff-Eisner, who also investigated this problem, attempted the separation by stating that the processes in which toxins are involved lead to the formation of antitoxins; processes in which endotoxins represent the effective agent lead to hypersensitivity. However, experience with tetanus immunization is at variance with this oversimplification.[23] The best evidence for the association of immunity with hypersensitiveness can be derived from work on vaccination.

In his early creative period von Pirquet attacked another problem in a field entirely unrelated to allergy which bears witness to his many-sided nature. In 1907 he published an article on the anodic hypersensitivity of infants which became of paramount importance in the investigation of infantile tetany. Here for the first time authentic values were established for the normal sensitivity of the peripheral nerves of infants. Von Pirquet found that in normal infants without tetany only the two closing contractions, cathodal and anodal, occur at an intensity of galvanic current below 5 milliamperes. At anodal opening, twitching which occurs below that intensity of the current indicates anodal hypersensitivity, characteristic of tetany. The next step is cathodal hypersensitivity, which is the occurrence of twitching at intensity values below 5 milliamperes for the cathode. Occurrence of anodal-opening twitching below that intensity of current, in the absence of cathodal-opening twitching and cathodal-closing

[21] Sitzung der K. K. Gesellschaft der Arzte, 22. Feb. 1907. *Wien. klin. Wchnschr.* No. 9, p. 272.

[22] "Allergie," *München. med. Wchnschr.* 53 (1906): 1457.

[23] Von Behring sensed this contradiction when he interpreted as a "paradoxical reaction" the death of animals highly immunized against tetanus and reinjected with small amounts of toxin.

tetanus, is characteristic of a mild degree of hypersensitivity. The next degree of tetanic hypersensitivity is shown by the occurrence of cathodal-closing tetanus or an opening twitching with a current of less than 5 milliamperes.[24]

When the investigation was made von Pirquet was still an assistant in the *Kinderklinik*. Escherich considered the results to be highly significant at a time when rickets was a common disease and tetany a frequent complication, and he emphasized the practical application of the discovery in diagnosis. Later, when head of the pediatric department in Vienna, von Pirquet had each child examined routinely with galvanic current when admitted to the infants' ward and monthly during the stay.

In those early years of his medical career von Pirquet produced in rapid succession a series of fundamental contributions to medical knowledge. Many were dramatic discoveries; all represented valuable scientific research. A brilliant investigator, the wise counsel and encouragement of Escherich, youthful enthusiasm spurred by the knowledge of success—all combined to make those formative years in Vienna the most consistently productive period of von Pirquet's life.

[24] "Die anodische Übererregbarkeit der Säuglinge," *Wien. med. Wchnschr.* 57 (1907): 14.

V

Important Medical Discoveries

Four of von Pirquet's most significant discoveries, which are interrelated and stem from the same chain of thought, will be discussed together—namely, the concepts of serum sickness, incubation time, allergy, and the tuberculin test which became known throughout the world as Pirquet's reaction. The tuberculin test was a natural outgrowth from the theory of allergy. Von Pirquet himself called it an allergy test.

Incubation Time, Serum Sickness, and Allergy

When not quite twenty-nine years old, Clemens von Pirquet deposited with the Imperial Academy of Sciences in Vienna a sealed envelope containing a statement on the theory of infectious diseases. He was at that time an unknown resident at the *Kinderklinik*, but so sure of himself and of the far-reaching significance of his discovery that he prepared a preliminary report to establish priority. Five years later he requested that the envelope be opened and the contents read. This was done at a meeting of the Academy's Division for Mathematics and Natural Sciences, and the action was recorded: "Dr. Clemens Freiherr von Pirquet of Vienna sent a sealed, written statement entitled 'On the Theory of Infectious Diseases' to the meeting of April 2, 1903 for the safeguarding of priority. Upon the wish of the author it was opened on February 13, 1908 in the presence of an academic commission and presented to the Division."

The contents of the sealed statement are translated here.

There are many spontaneous or experimental diseases of external origin in which the moment of entry of the foreign body, whether infective or intoxicative, is separated by an interval of time from the onset of the signs of illness. That interval is the stage of incubation of the disease.

As far as it has been possible to generalize until now, such illnesses resemble one another so closely that it is possible to take a uniform view of them.

Facsimile of first page of von Pirquet's statement
establishing priority on the theory of infectious diseases.

The manifestations of disease begin suddenly; they consist of fever, other constitutional symptoms (1–6), and exanthemata (1, 4–6), as numbered in brackets below. They are accompanied by a sudden decrease in the number of leukocytes, which increase again during the stage of incubation.

The next stage is the appearance in the blood stream of antibodies which bring about specific reactions with the causative foreign body (1–3). The antibodies disappear, but the ability persists to reproduce the entire process within a shorter time on a renewed attack by the foreign body (1–4).

Observations of the following conditions are used in drawing those conclusions:

I. After subcutaneous injection of foreign substances of animal or bacterial origin, which are incapable of multiplication

   A. Manifestations after *injection of serum in human beings* (observations in *St. Anna's Kinderspital; cf.* papers on antitoxic sera)   [1]

   B. The same in *animals* (von Dungern, Hamburger and Moro, and others). The manifestations after injection of tuberculin apply here.   [2]

II. After incorporation of living bacteria with their metabolic products: manifestations during the *immunization of horses with the streptococcus of scarlet fever*   [3]

III. After introduction, without their metabolic products, of infective organisms capable of multiplication

   A. Experimental

      In vaccination (observations of Bohn, Filatow, Sobotka, and others, confirmed in *St. Anna's Kinderspital*)   [4]

   B. In acute infectious diseases: variola, morbilli (measles)   [5, 6]

Hence I conclude:

1. The length of the incubation time depends not only upon the foreign body, but also upon the organism in question.

2. The manifestations of disease appear at the moment when the antibodies formed in the organism begin to react with the causative foreign body.

3. The acquired immunity, which persists, lies in the ability of the organism to produce the antibodies more rapidly than before, and there is a corresponding shortening of incubation time. Hence there follows a clinical difference between antitoxic (Group I) and antibacterial (Group III) immunity in that the reaction, the earlier it appears, is stronger in the former and weaker in the latter.

I intend to publish in collaboration with Dr. Bela Schick the observations upon which the above conclusions are based.

The ideas expressed by von Pirquet had originated earlier with other scientists, but it was he who recognized hitherto unexplained phenomena as the result of altered states of reactivity within the organism. It is common knowledge that the first attack of various infectious diseases is followed by a lasting immunity. The mechanism of that specific immunity was first observed by Roux in 1889 when he injected the blood serum of a rabbit, artificially immunized against staphylococci, into untreated animals and thereby transferred the resistance. Then followed the discovery that the blood serum of animals which had been immunized against the toxin of tetanus or diphtheria would neutralize the corresponding toxin both *in vivo* and *in vitro*. During the following decade it became apparent that the parenteral introduction of various complex substances caused new properties to be produced in the animal's blood serum. Such serum may specifically clump (agglutinate) small particles, such as bacteria or red blood cells, dissolve them, precipitate colloids from solutions, or have various other effects. The substances which produced such effects in the animal body received the name of antigens, and the agent upon which the specific response of the blood serum depended was called an antibody. Soon afterward it was observed not only that injection of an antigen produced antibodies, but also that a substance which was innocuous when first injected might on subsequent injection produce highly toxic effects.

The French physiologist Richet found in 1902 that the toxin of a sea urchin (*Echinoidea*) acted much more quickly and produced a stronger reaction if repeated injections were given at intervals of a few days. He assumed that the toxin had two different properties, an immunizing or "prophylactic" fraction and a hypersensitizing or "anaphylactic" fraction, but did not recognize the association with serum sickness. The two substances have not been separated or their existence proved, but the term anaphylaxis has survived. Theobald Smith of Boston also observed in 1902 that guinea pigs, used for the standardization of diphtheria toxin, frequently succumbed when the injection of serum was repeated. L. Dienes of Boston, a bacteriologist, reported that Ehrlich became interested in the phenomenon while visiting Theobald Smith and persuaded Kolle, one of his associates, to study it.

Independent of these investigations, von Pirquet studied similar reactions by observing patients. At the end of 1902 he concluded that the existing theory of incubation time was incorrect and advanced his new theory that *a pathogenic agent causes signs of illness in the organism only when modified by the presence*

*of antibody; the incubation time is thus the time which elapses before
the formation of antibody.*

Application of the theory, for instance to smallpox vaccination,
led von Pirquet and Schick to observe the symptoms following
repeated injection of horse serum and formed the basis of their
work on serum sickness. They emphasized that the eruption of
serum sickness was not a local skin reaction but that all organs
were involved. They discovered the difference between accelerated
and immediate ability to react and pointed out the significance of
the latter for detecting that an illness had previously been experienced. Through the action of antibody-like substances a
foreign protein, in itself nontoxic, can acquire toxic properties
(apotoxin).

Serum sickness is a classical illustration of the fact that certain
well-known scientific phenomena can be misinterpreted for years
until a genius clarifies their significance. In the case of serum
sickness, full understanding was of particular importance to safe-
guard human life. Some of the details mentioned here were contained in Friedrich Blittersdorf's excellent history of the subject.[1]

Human disease was first treated with antitoxic serum from
an outside source in 1891. Kitasato, co-worker of von Behring,
injected 1.5 ml. of serum from a rabbit immunized against tetanus into a nine-day-old infant who was suffering from tetanus.
Wernicke carried out the first experiments with diphtheria antitoxin. No exact results were published but Wernicke stated in a
letter that amounts of sheep serum up to 50 ml. had been well
tolerated by children in the *Charité* in Berlin. In 1892, the case
history was reported in detail of a twenty-five-year-old German
employed as a groom who was treated for tetanus with the massive
total dose of 261 ml. of horse serum. On the eleventh day of treatment a violent, itching, urticaria-like skin rash was noticed, particularly on the thighs, which obviously were the sites of injection.
That seems to have been the first documented account in the
literature of a serum rash. Previously, however, after transfusions
with lamb's blood, urticaria and shock-like conditions had been
observed. Wernicke also noted urticaria during the serum treatment of diphtheria, but did not recognize the significance. The
serum had been obtained from dogs and he considered it entirely

[1] F. Blittersdorf, "Zur Geschichte der Serumkrankheit," *Sudhoff Arch. Gesch.
Med.* 36 (1952): 149. (Courtesy of Franz Steiner Verlag, Wiesbaden.)

harmless. Von Behring shared Wernicke's opinion and declared antitoxic sera to be as innocuous as sterile salt solution.

Nevertheless, in 1894 Lublinski reported a case of serum sickness accompanied by severe shock. That was the first mention in the literature of alarming complications, with high fever and unconsciousness. Other reports of untoward side effects followed rapidly, and by the end of 1895 all known complications of serum treatment had been enumerated: hemorrhages into the skin, severe gastrointestinal difficulties, rheumatoid manifestations, joint effusions, lymphadenopathy, edema of the face, paralysis of the arm, and distinct signs of shock with angina pectoris, vomiting, and urgency. The serum rash was described as urticaria-like, morbilliform or scarlatiniform, frequently resembling erythema exudativum multiforme, and occasionally looking like rubella.

The first fatality, reported in Germany in 1896, was particularly tragic because the diphtheria serum had not been administered for therapeutic purposes but only for prophylaxis. The victim was the two-year-old child of the pathologist Langerhans, discoverer of the islets in the pancreas named for him. The child died in typical shock, five minutes after the injection. The "case Langerhans" was discussed, both in the Berlin press and in the medical literature, in several highly polemic articles. Before the accident to the Langerhans child, fatalities had occurred elsewhere—in France, for instance, where in 1894 Roux had introduced serum treatment for diphtheria—but had not been reported in the literature. In those early days, serum sickness and the shock induced by the foreign protein were more severe and of longer duration than at present because the serum was not highly purified. The sensitizing influence of previously administered serum was not then known. Repeated therapeutic and prophylactic administration of serum was frequently mentioned in the medical literature, and the procedure was recommended.

The fatalities caused by serum sickness should be clearly distinguished from other fatal accidents in the history of medicine which result from human error. For example, before toxoids were given routinely for active immunization against diphtheria, mixtures of toxin with antitoxin were used. In a crèche in Baden near Vienna pure toxin was given, not neutralized by the admixture of antitoxin. Seven deaths resulted. (When the tragic mistake was discussed in the Supreme Council of Public Health in Vienna, von Pirquet tactfully advised postponement of active immunization against diphtheria until the safe toxoid procedure could be generally introduced.)

Another accident happened in Lübeck, Germany, during an attempt to immunize infants against tuberculosis; a considerable number died after they had been given by mouth a strain of virulent tubercle bacilli instead of the harmless Calmette-Guerin bacillus. Both disasters were due to mistakes made in the laboratory, which can happen as long as vaccines are prepared by fallible human beings. The underlying principle was not invalidated, however. Such mistakes should not be hushed up but should be explained to the public and to the news reporters. Otherwise a sound procedure may fall into ill repute.

The medical profession did not fully understand the nature of the untoward reactions. For a short time the antitoxin itself was considered to be the cause of serum sickness; then other properties of the animal serum were questioned, still rather vaguely. At one time or another the phenol content of the serum, a concomitant streptococcal infection, or an unsatisfactory technique of administration was blamed. The edema around the site of inoculation was attributed to lack of sterility and once was mistaken for an abscess and incised. Control experiments with untreated horse serum produced reactions like those which accompanied injection of diphtheria antitoxin, but the true and now familiar interpretation of serum sickness as a manifestation of hypersensitivity was not known for almost another decade. Blittersdorf described three fundamental discoveries made in 1903 which resolved the problem.

First, Arthus injected rabbits repeatedly with horse serum at six-day intervals. Manifestations of hypersensitivity, local or generalized, immediate or delayed, occurred after the fourth injection at the earliest, the interval depending upon whether the injection was subcutaneous or intravenous. Occurrence of the local sign known as the Arthus phenomenon was not linked to use of the same site for repeated injections, for it could follow a subcutaneous injection even though the earlier administration had been intraperitoneal. Intravenous administration of the serum—after previous subcutaneous or intraperitoneal injection—might precipitate an immediate reaction with sneezing, nervous excitement, and finally cessation of respiration; or, when sensitivity was low, there might be transitory shock followed by fatal cachexia after a few days of well-being. At the same time Arthus discovered the *principle of specificity*, which meant that the phenomenon could be produced by repeatedly injecting cow's milk into rabbits, but that the rabbits did not react to injection of horse serum after the milk treatment.

The great value of this discovery lies in Arthus' recognition of the principle that increased sensitivity follows repeated injection of a foreign protein which is primarily nontoxic; he speaks of *liquides albumineux*. He recognized the relationship of increased sensitivity to the anaphylaxis of Portier and Richet.[2]

Arthus published his discovery on June 25, 1903. Nine days later, Pirquet and Schick's preliminary note on the theory of incubation time appeared,[3] followed by more detailed conclusions. Their classic monograph on serum sickness was published two years later, and at about the same time von Pirquet presented a paper on this subject at the 77th assembly of the Society of German Natural Scientists and Physicians in Meran.[4] A fundamental biological law emerged, and for the first time some of the adverse effects previously called toxic serum effects, serum rash, antitoxin eruption or—by the French—serotherapeutic accidents, were summarized under the new name of serum sickness. Meanwhile, general interest in the adverse effects had diminished even before the signs and symptoms had been satisfactorily explained. Arthus explained anaphylaxis as essentially the result of repeated injections of horse serum;[5] but the concept of von Pirquet and Schick was focused on the "time factor"—the interval between the first injection and the onset of serum sickness. Von Pirquet had observed an accelerated reaction in two children and recognized that the incubation time preceding signs of hypersensitivity was shorter after each repetition of the injection. Further study suggested the theory that serum sickness is induced by the "collision of antigen and antibody"[6] (Figs. 8-10).

[2] "De l'action anaphylactique de certain venins," *Soc. de Biol.* (1902): 170.

[3] "Zur Theorie der Inkubationszeit," *Wien. klin. Wchnschr.* 16 (1903): 1244. (With B. Schick.)

[4] "Neuere Beobachtungen über die Serumkrankheit," *Jahrbuch f. Kinderheilk.* 62 (1905): 537.

[5] M. Arthus, "Injections répétées de sérum de cheval chez le lapin," *Compt. rendu Soc. de Biol.* 50 (1903): 20.

[6] *Die Serumkrankheit* (Vienna: Franz Deuticke, 1905). (With B. Schick. Translated into English by Schick in 1927.)

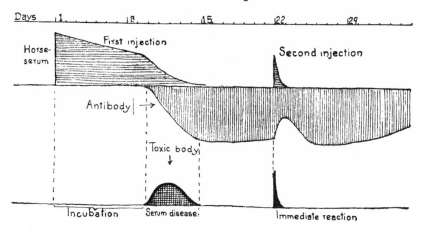

Fig. 8. Effects of horse serum in man. *From:* "Allergy," *Arch. Int. Med.* 7 (1911): 383. (Courtesy of American Medical Association, Chicago.)

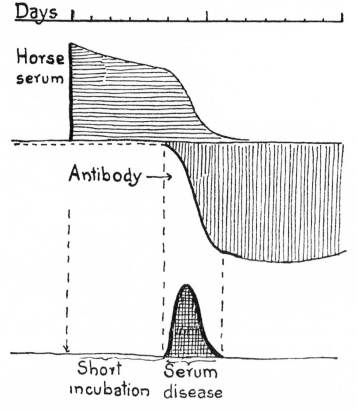

Fig. 9. Accelerated serum disease in a rabbit. *From:* "Allergy," *Arch. Int. Med.* 7 (1911): 383. (Courtesy of American Medical Association, Chicago.)

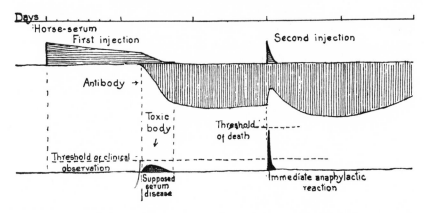

Fig. 10. Effects of horse serum in guinea pigs or rabbits. *From:* "Allergy," *Arch. Int. Med.* 7 (1911): 383. (Courtesy of American Medical Association, Chicago.)

Another finding of von Pirquet and Schick deserves particular attention: "This peculiarity of reacting more quickly to the introduction of a pathogenic substance can be experimentally transmitted to an organism as yet untreated by means of serum from an organism which has already experienced the disease in question." In each of three rabbits, 10 ml. of horse serum was injected into the skin of the abdomen; after twenty-four hours, when absorption was complete but active antibody formation could not yet be assumed, two of the animals each received into the ear vein 2 ml. of anti-horse serum from a sensitized rabbit, and the third rabbit received 2 ml. of normal serum from a nonsensitized rabbit. There was no trace of reaction in the third animal, but one of the two rabbits which had received sensitized serum displayed the typical edema and the other had slight edema of the ear.[7]

The theory that an antigen-antibody reaction was involved received strong support from the third important discovery made in 1903, when Hamburger and Moro found precipitating antibodies in the blood during serum sickness[8] (Fig. 11). After further study, undertaken jointly with Hamburger, von Pirquet left the question open. Later he rejected the possibility that the precipitin could have any identification with the antibody of serum sickness.

[7] "Überempfindlichkeit und beschleunigte Reaktion," *München. med. Wchnschr.* 53 (1906): 66. (With B. Schick.)

[8] F. Hamburger, and E. Moro, "Ueber die biologisch nachweisbaren Veränderungen des menschlichen Blutes nach der Seruminjektion," *Wien. klin. Wchnschr.* 16 (1903): 445.

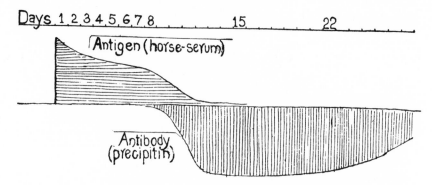

Fig. 11. Formation of precipitin in rabbits after injection of horse serum. *From:* "Allergy," *Arch. Int. Med.* 7 (1911): 383. (Courtesy of American Medical Association, Chicago.)

The failure of clinical manifestations to coincide with the demonstration of antibodies, either *in vitro* or in experimental animals, is still a valid reason for refusing to identify precipitin as the antibody specific to serum sickness. As late as 1933, Coca completely rejected the antigen-antibody explanation and interpreted serum sickness as a "specifically altered reactivity of the protoplasm."[9] His opinion, however, found few supporters; there was never serious disagreement with von Pirquet and Schick's interpretation of serum sickness.

In 1906, von Pirquet's concept of allergy established the bridge between immunity and hypersensitivity. The following year brought the discovery, through the work of Besredka and Steinhardt, of the antianaphylactic state after the occurrence of shock.[10] Still more important was Ulrich Friedemann's demonstration that acquired hypersensitivity could be passively transferred.[11] Friedemann's work proved an observation which the findings of von Pirquet and Schick, at that time almost forgotten, had rendered more than probable—namely, that hypersensitivity is conditioned by an antibody circulating in the serum. Von Pirquet explained this process by saying that when horse serum is first injected into a rabbit, antibodies are present. After several weeks, when a second injection is given (Fig. 12), the horse serum

[9] A. F. Coca, "A Critical Review of Investigations of Allergic Diseases," *Ergebn. Hyg.* 14 (1933): 538.

[10] A. Besredka and E. Steinhardt, "De l'anaphylaxie et de l'anti-anaphylaxie. Vis-à-vis du sérum de cheval," *Ann. Inst. Pasteur* 21 (1907): 117.

[11] U. Friedemann, "Ueber passive Ueberempfindlichkeit," *München. med. Wchnschr.* 54 (1907): 2414.

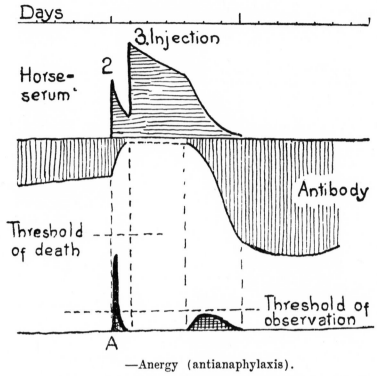

—Anergy (antianaphylaxis).

Fig. 12. Experiment on rabbits several weeks after the first injection of horse serum. *From:* "Allergy," *Arch. Int. Med.* 7 (1911): 383. (Courtesy of American Medical Association, Chicago.)

immediately unites with the existing antibodies, producing a toxic action and acute symptoms. If a third injection is given twenty-four hours later, no symptoms occur.

Subsequent studies on anaphylaxis have been based on the clinical and experimental foundations laid during that era of research. Investigators try in particular to clarify the nature of the antigen and the antibody, the interrelationship of the individual immunological phenomena, and the mechanism by which allergic signs and symptoms are produced. Invention of the electron microscope, ultracentrifuge, and electrophoresis apparatus established possibilities for further research, the fruits of which can already be recognized. The entire study started with von Pirquet's brilliant ideas and lightning flashes of insight.

Without any preconceived opinions, von Pirquet began to study changes in the ability of the human organism to react.

Existing terminology seemed to him inadequate and he suggested the term allergy. The highlights of these findings on allergy are given in his own words:

The connection between immunity and hypersensitivity appears to me most evident from experience with vaccination for smallpox. A recently revaccinated individual appears to be hypersensitive when compared with one vaccinated for the first time because he reacts much more quickly to the infection. At the same time he is protected, for the vaccinial process is characterized by an insignificant local reaction and all constitutional signs are absent.

Immunity and hypersensitivity can thus be closely related but the words contradict one another; their combination is very strained. The concept of immunity is carried over from the time when hypersensitivity was not known . . . . We need a new, more general term, devoid of bias, to denote the change experienced by an organism from its contact with an organic poison, whether live or inanimate. The reaction toward a given toxin of an individual who has not previously been in contact with it differs from the reaction of an individual who has. Such a changed reaction is shown by a vaccinated individual toward calf lymph, by the syphilitic toward the syphilis virus, by the tuberculous toward tuberculin, and by the individual injected with horse serum toward horse serum. The treated individual is far from being insensitive. All that can be said is that his ability to react has changed.

For this general concept of a change in ability to react, I suggest the term *allergy*. Allos means "other" and hence a deviation from the original state or from normal behavior, as in allorhythmia and allotropism.

The vaccinated, the tuberculous, and the individual injected with horse serum become allergic toward the respective foreign body. On the other hand, a foreign substance which induces the organism to react in a changed manner to its single or repeated introduction into the body is an *allergen*. The word is modeled on the term antigen (Detre-Deutsch) in a manner highly discordant with the laws of philology.[12] An antigen is a substance which is capable of producing antibodies; the concept of an allergen includes, in addition to the antigens, numerous protein substances which do not promote formation of antibodies but cause hypersensitivity. . . . All organisms causing infectious diseases which are followed by immunity are allergens; so are the toxins of mosquitoes and of bees, since they induce manifestations of hypo- or hypersensitivity.

[12] Schadewaldt ("Die geschichtliche Bedeutung der Pädiatrie für die Entwicklung der Allergie," *Medizinische*, 14 [1959]: 681) criticized von Pirquet's choice of the term allergy on a purely linguistic basis. He claimed that the Greek word *ergon* from which it was derived means first of all work or activity, whereas allergy is used to express a readiness to react that is a passive state or condition.

For the same reason, we can include the pollen causing hay fever (Wolff-Eisner), the urticaria-producing substances of strawberries and of crustaceans, and probably also a series of organic substances giving rise to idiosyncrasy.

The term immunity should be limited to those states in which the introduction of a foreign substance does not result in any clinical reaction. Thus there exists a complete absence of sensitivity, which may be conditioned by natural immunity (alexins), by antitoxins (active or passive immunity, as against diphtheria or tetanus), or by some kind of adaptation to the toxin (Wassermann and Citron).[13]

Many years later the editor of a Vienna medical journal requested von Pirquet to write a short article reviewing the history of allergy. This he did in 1927 and drew additional conclusions.

Jenner's inoculation against smallpox provides the best way of studying the course of an artificially induced infection in the human subject. I studied that disease thoroughly and came to the following conclusions: a change in the ability of an organism to react is clearly proved by the clinical signs after vaccination and revaccination. The local reaction in a primary take is distinguished in its time and pattern from that seen after revaccination, with its early reaction and accelerated local reaction. Immunity in the sense of insensitivity occurs only in the months immediately following an initial vaccination.

The following conclusions I consider as scientifically established: (1) The early reaction, or reaction of immunity, is a meeting between antibodies already existing and the newly reintroduced toxin. (2) The local symptoms constitute two separate processes—the growth of the causative organism and the formation of antibodies within the body. (3) The accelerated area reaction is an accelerated formation of antibodies.

These new conclusions culminate in the concept that inflammatory manifestations occur through the action of antibodies; what has long been called a "reaction" of the organism is to be understood as active formation of antibodies. Until now only the termination of the vaccinial or variolar process has been regarded as the result of antibody formation.

Wide dissemination of the variolar skin rash takes place during the phase when general antibodies appear. The early reaction of allergy following cutaneous inoculation is of diagnostic value in vaccinia, variola, tuberculosis, and probably in a series of other infectious diseases.[14]

[13] "Allergie," *München. med. Wchnschr.* 53 (1906): 1457. (Courtesy of Verlag J. F. Lehmann, Munich.)

[14] "Zur Geschichte der Allergie," *Wien. med. Wchnschr.* 23 (1927): 745. (Courtesy of Brüder Hollinek, Vienna.)

As recently as 1967, Holborow of Great Britain commented that the modern approach in immunology began with von Pirquet, who made the fundamental distinction between immunity and hypersensitivity from a biological rather than a clinical point of view. Von Pirquet recognized at the turn of the century that "a common biological process of specific sensitization" was present irrespective of clinical response. In the succeeding decades most investigators have continued to follow his approach and have placed greatest emphasis on the problem of hypersensitivity.[15]

The Tuberculin Test

The same train of thought appeared in von Pirquet's first presentation of his cutaneous tuberculin test. On May 8, 1907, he told the Medical Society of Berlin that his investigations had originated when he distinguished between the reaction following a first vaccination against smallpox and the so-called early reaction after revaccination, due to the effect of antibodies. "This principle can be applied to other diseases. If a tuberculous child is inoculated, not with cowpox vaccine but with tuberculin, a

[15] E. J. Holborow, "An ABC of Modern Immunology. I. Links between the Old and the New," *Lancet* 1 (Apr. 15, 1967): 833.

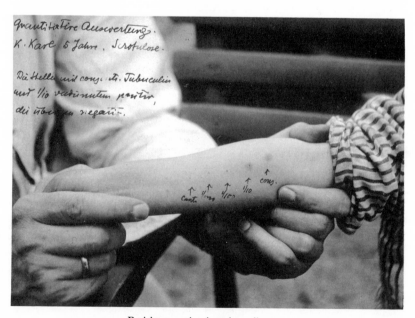

Positive reaction in tuberculin test.

small papule occurs at the site of the inoculation which is light red at the beginning, gradually becomes dark red, and fades within eight days . . . ."[16] A month later he described the test to the pediatric section of the medical society in Vienna, and publication followed.[17]

Several other papers about the tuberculin test were published thereafter.

A positive reaction to the tuberculin test signifies that the individual has been in contact with the tubercle bacillus. It is not possible, however, to conclude directly from that finding in what stage of tuberculosis the individual is; the disease may be either active and progressive or inactive. The younger the individual, the more probable it is that the process is malign, for we know that latent, inactive tuberculosis is rarely found at autopsy in the first years of life. A positive reaction is therefore of grave significance at that time of life and particularly during infancy; in an adult, on the other hand, no conclusion can be drawn in relation to prognosis.[18] In such an instance, in the absence of signs in the lungs, a positive reaction is probably to be attributed to a few small foci in the lymph nodes. A negative tuberculin reaction in a healthy small child indicates the absence of tubercular changes. In older children and adults a negative reaction rules out only active tuberculosis because old foci, such as caseous lymph nodes, do not always produce a positive reaction. In cachectic individuals we cannot draw any conclusion from a negative test, since a positive reaction disappears in the last stage of tuberculosis. It disappears also in many instances during the last ten days of miliary tuberculosis and tuberculous meningitis. I believe that diagnosis by allergy in general, particularly through the use of the cutaneous tuberculin test, will be capable of expanding considerably diagnostic possibilities for the general practitioner.

The cutaneous reaction in tuberculosis has many advantages compared with other allergy tests; I am of the opinion that it will remain superior to the ophthalmic test. In consequence of my publications, Wolff-Eisner and later Calmette tried applying tuberculin to the conjunctiva; a

[16] "Tuberkulindiagnose durch cutane Impfung." Sessions of Berliner medizinischen Gesellschaft, May 8 and 15, 1907. *Berlin. klin. Wchnschr.* 20 (May 20, 1907).

[17] "Die Allergieprobe zur Diagnose der Tuberkulose im Kindesalter," *Wien. med. Wchnschr.* 57 (1907): 1369. A second paper, "Der diagnostische Wert der Kutanen Tuberkulinreaktion bei der Tuberkulose des Kindesalters auf Grund von 100 Sektionen," was published in *Wien. klin. Wchnschr.* 20 (1907): 1123.

[18] As usual, the pathologist had the last word. Ghon, who found the primary focus in the lungs of children, and for whom the tubercle was named, was pathologist in Vienna at that time. He established the diagnostic value of the cutaneous tuberculin test on the basis of one hundred postmortem examinations.

tuberculous individual responds with conjunctivitis. Vallel used the same test in cattle, where it may be more practical than the cutaneous reaction. In human subjects I would not recommend it, since the manifestations of the reaction give rise to unpleasant sensations and cannot be checked so objectively.

In childhood the allergy test for tuberculosis is important in prevention as well as diagnosis. In day nurseries, hospitals, or orphanages it is now possible to segregate the tuberculous children and thus protect the others against infection. Further, we shall learn to recognize the early stages of tuberculosis and to introduce adequate treatment before serious localized manifestations have appeared. In that sense the allergy test will have therapeutic value as well.

Based on statistical observations of tubercular infection in childhood obtained by means of the tuberculin skin reaction, I made further studies, in collaboration with Schnürer, of allergy tests in bovines.[19] As the simplest way of eliminating tuberculosis from a herd of cattle, the conjunctival reaction is recommended as a screening test. With an unquestionably positive result the animal is considered tuberculous; when the result is equivocal or negative, the subcutaneous test should be carried out. [20]

Von Pirquet's mention of the value of the tuberculin test in the prevention of tuberculosis points to a function which may be of even greater significance than its diagnostic value in individual patients. In the majority of cases, a positive tuberculin reaction in a preschool child suggests an intrafamilial source of infection. When an older child has a positive reaction the source may be extrafamilial, such as a teacher or a family visitor. Through an awareness of the source, tuberculin-negative children can be protected from infection. The possibility of cross-infection from child to child is slight. The most dangerous contact is the adolescent or adult with open tuberculosis.

At the end of 1907, Preisich of Budapest pointed out a significant reason why a test might be negative even in an individual with tuberculosis, and von Pirquet studied the problem carefully. He discovered that *during measles* tubercular children lose the capacity to react to tuberculin for about one week. This phenomenon seems consistent with the finding that the tubercular process frequently spreads during measles. A positive tuberculin

---

[19] "Allergie bei Tuberkulose der Rinder," *Monatshefte f. prakt. Tierh.*, Stuttgart, 19 (1908): 405. (With Schnürer.)

[20] "Allergie-Diagnostik," *Therap. Monatshefte*, 21 (1907): 555. (Courtesy of Springer–Verlag, Heidelberg.)

test can be utilized in the differential diagnosis of a doubtful skin rash.

Discussing the subject before the Chicago Medical Society on October 14, 1908, he described his method of applying the test:

The skin of the forearm is scrubbed with ether; then two drops of un-diluted old tuberculin are dropped about four inches distant from each other. Then, with a vaccinating lancet, the point of which has the form of a small chisel, a superficial circular scarification is made between the two drops (for the control of the traumatic redness following the small scarification). Finally, the same scarification is made inside of the two drops; a few fibers of cotton are put on the drops so that they will not flow. After five minutes the cotton is taken off. No dressing is applied. The papule is examined after twenty-four and forty-eight hours. It is considered as positive when the tuberculin scarifications are clearly different from the control places, but the inflammatory reactive area must measure at least 1/6 of an inch (5 mm.).[21]

In several studies subsequently carried out in Baltimore von Pirquet elaborated quantitative details of the tuberculin test and made observations on cutaneous reactions in general. While in Breslau he worked out more details of smallpox vaccination.

Study of the skin rash in measles in 1913 marked the end of von Pirquet's first creative period—the immune-biological. All of the theories which he established in his youth, unlike many theories in medicine which have survived only briefly, are as valid today as when they were formulated. He pointed out this fact himself, two years before he died.

When after many years I look back on my early work, I am happy to state that none of the conclusions which I then labeled as positive and reliable were false. The term serum sickness and the concepts of allergy and of antigen-antibody reaction have been generally accepted. The vast literature on those subjects which has since been published does not nullify the postulates and observations I made at that time. The finding of most practical importance, the cutaneous tuberculin test, is used by pediatricians all over the world with the same interpretation I devised years ago; and the diphtheria test discovered by my coworker, Bela Schick, has become a common tool of the medical profession. Both tests have rendered fundamental service in the understanding of tuberculosis and diphtheria.[22]

[21] "Frequency of Tuberculosis in Childhood," *J. Amer. Med. Assn.* 52 (1909): 675. (A week before, the J.A.M.A. had carried the notice of von Pirquet's move to Baltimore.)
[22] Von Pirquet, "Zur Geschichte der Allergie."

Von Pirquet's work stands on its own merit and an epilogue is scarcely needed. A brief but very perceptive summary was written in 1929, which places special emphasis on the tuberculin test.[23] For a considerable time after his death little progress was made in the field of allergy although, particularly in this country, allergy has become an independent specialty. The name of its discoverer is no longer associated with it, but the term allergic is widely used even in American slang.

Interest in von Pirquet's work waned when his clinical observations could not be reproduced in animals by injection of several protein antigens which produce abundant antibodies. The allergy process which he studied appears to have been related to antibody production yet somehow different. It has slowly been realized that immunity is a complex process, the different components of which may develop with unequal intensity. The component corresponding to infectious allergy remains so slight after treatment with protein antigens that it was not identified until 1930. Our understanding of the mechanism of immunity is still incomplete. Our experimental technique, although greatly improved, is still imperfect, but the way is much clearer now for continuing von Pirquet's work and for studying the development of the immune process in disease with its influence on clinical manifestations and on the progress of healing.

Recent clinical and experimental observations fully confirm von Pirquet's insight into the importance of infectious allergy. The use of antibiotics has helped to save children who fail to produce antibodies because of a hereditary defect (agammaglobulinemia). The development of allergy in these children and their reaction to vaccinia, measles, and tuberculosis are the same as in normal children. The course of clinical symptoms and the healing process often depend upon the development of allergy. The important relationship of allergy to circulating antibodies is indicated also in other conditions. The auto-immune diseases, of which the prototype is experimental encephalitis in animals produced by injection of brain substance, are probably the result of allergy. In addition, allergy explains the rejection of transplants and the great difference in effectiveness of vaccination with live or dead bacteria and viruses.

[23] W. R. Bett, "Some Paediatric Eponyms. I. Pirquet's Reaction," *Brit. J. Child. Dis.* 26 (1929): 276.

Recently Baar traced the progress of immunology over the years, stating that for a long time it was considered to be synonymous with serology. "The first indication that cells have a more essential role than giving up antibodies into the circulation was provided by the study of anaphylaxis and the hypersensitivity reactions." Transplants are known to be accepted if they are taken from the same individual, from an identical twin, or from highly inbred strains of animals. Although the rejection of homotransplants as a result of the massive accumulation of lymphocytes was studied by Leo Loeb, it was Medawar who proved that the rejection process is immunological. Characteristic of an immunological reaction is that a second transplant is rejected more rapidly than the first. Baar continued:

In other words, we have the same phenomenon as that described by Pirquet as allergy. This was defined as the altered reaction of an animal or human individual to an antigen with which it or he had a previous contact. The word allergy is nowadays frequently used as synonymous with hypersensitivity. However, in Pirquet's definition it comprised immunological resistance, accelerated reaction, immediate and delayed hypersensitivity, negative and positive anergy. Pirquet attempted to explain all these phenomena, particularly revaccination, tuberculin reaction and serum sickness on the lines of classical humoral immunology. However, we have learned of immunological phenomena like the rejection of transplants in which humoral antibodies play no role and delayed hypersensitivity cannot be transmitted by serum injection but in highly inbred animals by injection of a cell suspension from lymph nodes or spleen.

Lymphocytes are mainly responsible for cellular immunity without humoral antibodies. Baar stated aptly that it was a long way from Ehrlich and Pirquet to the new immunology of Medawar and Burnet.[24]

Recent findings on immunologic processes which pertain to problems of hypersensitivity were presented in Detroit at an international symposium. Sixty-five specialists from many countries presented their different viewpoints on allergy and dermatology, immunology, and allied sciences. Their survey of this rapidly expanding field gives the first comprehensive evidence for the

[24] H. S. Baar, "From Ehrlich-Pirquet to Medawar and Burnet. A Revolution in Immunology," *J. Maine Med. Assn.* 54 (1963): 209. (Courtesy of Brunswick Publishing Company, Brunswick, Maine.)

part played by serum complement in allergic responses, as well as a thorough discussion of diseases due to auto-antibodies, the effect of antibodies on cultured cells, and the effect of antigen-antibody complexes on the whole organism.[25] At about the same time, twenty-two experts on pediatric allergy contributed to a symposium in this field.[26]

All of these discussions bear witness to the enormous importance of the problem of hypersensitivity. Von Pirquet had recognized the nature of the immune process through his study of human diseases. Many decades later, experimental observations have caused the limelight to be focused once more upon his work, and his brilliant concepts are receiving the recognition which is their due. We may say of his achievements, as Schiller said of Kant: "When the kings build, there is work for the artisans." Thus those who follow a genius work over his data and amplify his ideas.

[25] J. H. Shaffer, G. A. LoGrippo, and M. W. Chase, eds., *Mechanisms of Hypersensitivity*, Henry Ford Hospital International Symposium (Boston: Little, Brown and Co., 1959).

[26] L. W. Hill, and H. L. Mueller, cons. eds., "Symposium on Pediatric Allergy," *Pediat. Clin. No. Amer.* 6 (1959): 655.

VI

Baltimore

In 1909, at the age of thirty-five, von Pirquet declined a tempting offer from the Pasteur Institute in Paris, choosing instead to become the first professor of pediatrics at The Johns Hopkins University in Baltimore. The invitation to work at the Pasteur Institute was especially flattering because it came from Roux himself, who proposed to create a position which would give von Pirquet freedom to advance his research. The confidence of such a renowned scientist was high tribute to a young man. Von Pirquet visited the Institute in February 1908 and was greatly interested in the prospect of an association. After returning to Vienna he considered the offer carefully. Here was excellent opportunity to carry out the experimental studies he had envisioned, but for their clinical application he needed authority to establish contact with patients. The concern, expressed in his letter to Roux, for a suitable hospital appointment suggests the primary reason for his final refusal.

The events leading to the Johns Hopkins offer and acceptance, which were significant both for von Pirquet and for the University, are documented in an exchange of letters.[1] Early in 1907, plans were being made to organize pediatrics as a special branch of medicine at Johns Hopkins. The following resolutions were adopted by the Board of Trustees on March 4, 1907:

1. That a professorship or associate professorship of pediatrics be established in the University, and that the position be filled as soon as possible in order that the incumbent might participate in the work of building and organizing the new children's hospital.
2. That a committee of three be appointed, to meet with a similar committee of hospital trustees, for the purpose of selecting a professor of pediatrics.

The President of the Board designated Messrs. Remsen, Randall, and Buckler to form this committee.

[1] This correspondence was made available through the kindness of Dr. Edwards A. Park, who obtained some of the material compiled by the late Dr. Alan Chesney for a history of Johns Hopkins Medical School and Hospital. I am also indebted to Dr. Samuel Amberg for information.

On March 19 the joint committee's recommendation was submitted to the Board of Trustees by the chairman, Dr. Rupert Morton:

At a meeting of the joint committee of the trustees of the Johns Hopkins Hospital and of the Johns Hopkins University held Monday, the 18th inst., it was

Resolved that the Medical Board of the Hospital and the Advisory Board of the Medical Faculty be requested by the joint committee of the trustees of the Johns Hopkins Hospital and the Johns Hopkins University to recommend to the joint committee a proper man to be appointed Professor or Associate Professor of Pediatrics in the Medical School of the University and Physician-in-Chief to the Harriet Lane Johnston Home for Invalid Children of Baltimore City.

While a suitable candidate for the newly created position was being sought, von Pirquet made a presentation in Paris of the studies which resulted in his discovery of the tuberculin test. His paper was the highlight of the meeting. Robert Koch was so thoroughly convinced of the tremendous potential of the test and so much impressed with the ability and personality of its originator that after the presentation he introduced von Pirquet to Sir William Osler as the man to head Johns Hopkins' Department of Pediatrics.

Von Pirquet visited the United States in 1908 and described his tuberculin test to a group attending the International Congress of Tuberculosis in Washington, D.C. Dr. William H. Welch was president of the Congress and he immediately invited von Pirquet to Baltimore to meet other members of the Johns Hopkins faculty. As a result, the invitation was issued in 1908. Acceptance was delayed by simultaneous consideration of Roux's proposal, and it was not until January 5, 1909, that Mr. Ira Remsen, President of the Board of Trustees of the University, sent von Pirquet official confirmation of his appointment:

DEAR SIR:

At a recent meeting of the Trustees of the Johns Hopkins University you were elected Professor of Pediatrics, at a salary of four thousand dollars per annum. A part of this salary is to be paid by the Harriet Lane Home for Children, which is to be under the general management of the Johns Hopkins Hospital. The remainder of the salary will be paid by the University. The date of the beginning of your service will be determined later.

Hoping that you will accept this offer, I remain

Von Pirquet accepted immediately in a letter which, although not dated, was obviously written in January:

DEAR SIR:

In reply to yours of January the 5th, I beg to say that I accept your offer with great pleasure.

I have already secured plans of some of the newest children's hospitals, so that I shall be able to help the Board of the Harriet Lane Home with at least a few good ideas.

I shall start on my journey next week and hope to be in Baltimore about the 11th or 12th of February, 1909.

Once more my best thanks for your trust in me, and with kindest regards to the Board of the Johns Hopkins University.

And so he became the first head of an independent pediatric department at The Johns Hopkins Medical School. Previously this specialty had been under the administrative direction of the Department of Internal Medicine. The appointment was not full-time, but permitted private practice. In addition, as physician-in-chief of the Harriet Lane Home, von Pirquet took part in planning both the amphitheater and the new hospital. Such planning was not well suited to his talents, perhaps because it required too much attention to detail. Whatever the reason, the design of the amphitheater did not receive general approval. The building was completed before the discovery was made that no one had thought to provide seating. When this omission was brought to von Pirquet's attention, he quipped that at least if the students remained standing there would be little danger of their going to sleep during lectures.

Von Pirquet joined a distinguished faculty. Among his contemporaries were Lewellys F. Barker (Osler's successor), medicine; William S. Halsted, surgery; H. M. Hurd, superintendent of the hospital and professor of psychiatry; Howard A. Kelly, gynecology; J. W. Williams, obstetrics; William H. Welch, pathology; F. P. Mall, anatomy; William H. Howell, physiology; J. J. Abel, pharmacology; and W. Jones, physiologic chemistry. Other associates were Samuel Amberg, associate professor of pediatrics and later one of the leading pediatricians at the Mayo Clinic; J. H. Mason Knox and R. A. Wiguard, who belonged to the old guard of the department. Thus three (Halsted, Kelly, and Welch) of the four who appear in the famous painting by Sargent were still at the University; Osler left Johns Hopkins before von Pirquet's appointment took effect.

Welch's support of von Pirquet's candidacy was the beginning of a long friendship. The curriculum vitae prepared when von Pirquet was being considered for the professorship of pediatrics was in Welch's handwriting. In addition to listing degrees, positions, and publications, it contained the following statement:

Dr. von Pirquet, besides being well trained in the diagnosis and treatment of diseases of children, has made important contributions to medical knowledge through his original research work. His name is best known in connection with the so-called cutaneous method of diagnosing tuberculosis (and the paper he read upon the subject at the International Congress of Tuberculosis in Washington was listened to with great interest and discussed by many of the scientists present). One of his most important contributions is that which deals with the so-called serum disease, which is met with in a few cases after treatment with antitoxic serum of patients suffering from diphtheria. Dr. von Pirquet also published an important monograph upon vaccination and revaccination, in which he described many hitherto unobserved phenomena in connection with ordinary vaccination against smallpox. His studies upon the processes of immunity have led him to an interesting conception regarding the phenomenon known as hypersensitivity, and he has set out his views in full in a special monograph on the subject in which he deals with what he calls *Allergie*.

Prof. von Pirquet is a brother-in-law of Prof. von Eiselsberg, the distinguished Vienna surgeon. Though a member of the Austrian aristocracy, Prof. von Pirquet has a liking for the democratic tendencies of the American people, and those who have met him speak enthusiastically of the attractiveness of his personality.

Von Pirquet had great respect for Welch, and kept in his study a picture showing Welch on horseback in China against the background of the tombs of the Ming Dynasty. After his retirement, Welch's interest in the history of medicine brought him to Vienna each year, where he visited the Institute of History of Medicine at the University. His last visit with von Pirquet was in 1927.

The private and social life of the von Pirquets in Baltimore had no features of special note. Their friends were found mostly among the University faculty and the trustees of The Johns Hopkins Hospital and The Harriet Lane Home. Von Pirquet established a journal club in pediatrics for members of his department, and their meetings were held at his home. The department members also met there on other occasions. Rowntree, who visited von Pirquet both in Vienna and in Baltimore, called him "a most charming and remarkable man, tall, handsome, affable, and lovable. He wore glasses and a most becoming mustache. He was a fascinating speaker with a magnetic personality, a brilliant scientist, a first-class executive, and one of Europe's shining lights in medical science. He was the first to center medical attention on allergies." He stated that the von Pirquets were very popular in Baltimore and "set up a veritable menage which his salary could not support, so after a brief stay they returned to Europe."[2]

During the Baltimore period von Pirquet did not produce any outstanding work. Observers not familiar with the cyclic pattern of his creative periods may attribute the standstill to the demands and pressures of the new position and environment, to being involved in the building and organizing of the new children's hospital, or to lecturing in a language other than his mother tongue. However, from my own observation of the later period of his life I have concluded that no outside pressure would have been permitted to interfere if an inner drive had moved him to attack a new problem which he himself considered worth his all-out, total devotion. During such drives he would brush aside nonessentials, let his associates deal with the daily routine, and concentrate on his important work. This was the secret of his ability to complete some of his masterpieces within a surprisingly short time and to reach the heart of an investigative problem with brilliant thoroughness and the assiduity characteristic of a genius. The keynote in his creative periods was ability to recognize which things were most important. Men in leading positions often deem it their duty to handle the minutiae themselves and are unable to delegate such noncreative activities of their professional life as committee meetings, writing reports (which end in the wastepaper basket), or answering empty questionnaires. Not so von Pirquet. His timing was most economic; in the Vienna period he was a master in sharing the administrative duties of a great institution with his seven assistants. He was never in a hurry and had time for everybody and everything, particularly his own work. The balance of time was always positive for him. It was probably not the duties of the new position which prevented creative work.

[2] L. G. Rowntree, *Amid Masters of Twentieth Century Medicine* (Springfield, Illinois: C. C Thomas, 1958). (Courtesy of Charles C Thomas, publisher, Springfield.)

The Baltimore interlude was rather a true standstill. With the exception of one piece of investigation, von Pirquet's scientific publications in Baltimore were based almost entirely on his previous studies in Vienna.

At a Conference on the Prevention of Infant Mortality held in New Haven on November 11, 1909, von Pirquet discussed the frequency of tuberculosis in infancy on the basis of postmortem reports from Berlin, Vienna, and New York. In the second year of life, 40 per cent of deaths in Vienna and 39 per cent in New York were due to tuberculosis. He stated that this tremendous incidence had only recently been recognized because the clinical symptoms in infants take different forms, unlike the clear picture of pulmonary tuberculosis in adults.

The first form of tuberculosis in infants, called chronic tuberculosis of the visceral glands, is very often mistakenly looked upon as gastrointestinal marasmus. Without showing any signs on the outside of the body, the children gradually lose in weight and die after a few months. In the post mortem examination you will find a tuberculous condition and caseation of nearly all the glands of the lungs, of the peritoneum and mesentery. . . . Sometimes the post mortem examination shows besides this, tuberculous knots in the brain, bones, spleen, liver, and kidneys. The second form resembles more the tuberculosis in adults. . . . In the post mortem examination one finds, besides a tuberculosis of the bronchial glands, a lobular pneumonia of tuberculous character, very often combined with cavities. A third form comprises the cases of caseous pneumonia which also give very definite lung symptoms on percussion and auscultation, whereas the cough is sometimes lacking. The last form, which is more common than the others, is miliary tuberculosis, which is characterized on post mortem examination by the great number of very small tubercles spread over nearly all organs. Among the symptoms of the miliary form, the brain affection, tuberculous meningitis, nearly always predominates; that is, pressure is exerted by the cerebrospinal fluid, largely produced within the brain sinuses, through the presence of miliary tubercles. In fewer cases of miliary tuberculosis, the symptoms of the lungs prevail; we find a subacute bronchitis with high fever, and a marked swelling of the spleen, again a form in which tuberculosis is often not recognized.

Von Pirquet discussed only the fatal forms of the disease because in the first year of life nearly every such infection led to death. Since 1909 the situation has changed as a result of successful treatment. What has not changed is the condition of children between the ages of six and fourteen, who often become infected without showing any clinical symptoms.

In cases of this kind, tuberculosis is localized in the lymph nodes, and does not spread over the whole body. In infancy the power of localization of tuberculosis does not yet seem to be developed. An incipient state of tuberculosis is suspected by a gradual decrease in weight without any signs of a disease of the bowels or the skin, or of any other acute infection. In some cases it is suggested by a difficulty in breathing, which appears especially as a slight tracheal snoring during the night, a symptom due to the enlargement of the glands near the division of the trachea. In other cases symptoms are seen on the skin, in the bones, especially an enlargement of the fingers and toes, subcutaneous tuberculous gummas, and lately attention has been turned to various small eruptions on the skin which are called tuberculides. In all these cases the diagnosis is best established by the different kinds of tuberculin tests, especially my cutaneous test.

He raised the question of the entrance portal of the infection. It had been proven that tuberculosis is seldom congenital.

. . . we find in nearly every case of tuberculous infants another person in the neighborhood who has an open tuberculosis. Whether the infection is directly through droplets containing tuberculous germs coughed out by the infected person and then breathed in by the child, or by bacilli taken in from the dust of the room in which tuberculous sputum has dried out, is a question which has not yet been decided. In comparison with the danger of infection from other human beings in the neighborhood, that of infection through tuberculous milk is probably rather small. Still, the milk of cows with tuberculous udders very often contains tubercle bacilli, and we must consider it dangerous, and therefore remove all tuberculous cows from farms that supply milk for babies; if this is not done, or if we do not know the condition of the milk, then it must be boiled.

The most important way to prevent tuberculosis in infants is, however, to be careful that the baby does not come in contact with anyone who is likely to have tuberculosis of the lungs. We can ascertain almost with certainty that tuberculosis can be stamped out as a whole if this were possible socially, because in one instance it has been successfully carried out. In cattle, which are infected in a similar way as human beings, the disease was almost gotten rid of by adopting the system of Bang. It is carried out as follows: All cattle in one farm are tested with tuberculin, those which do not react are sent to a new farm. All calves which are born of tuberculous mothers are immediately separated from the mother and receive milk only after it has been boiled. Afterward they are sent to the healthy farm. After a number of years there are no more cattle in the infected farm and no tuberculous cases in the new farm. We cannot apply that system to humanity, except in orphan asylums, because it would interfere with our family relations, but still we can make people understand that a nursling is no toy for its relatives, and especially sick relatives, and that parents who have an open tuberculosis do better to apply as much caution as possible in kissing the child or coughing in its presence.

Von Pirquet concluded by saying: "America is now realizing the danger of tuberculosis, and I hope it will also realize the importance of raising a healthy generation by keeping it free from that dreadful disease." In the discussion which followed, Dr. Thomas Morgan Rotch of Boston spoke most enthusiastically about the value of the Pirquet skin test in early detection of tuberculosis in children, and added:

What Dr. von Pirquet has done already will make his name go down to posterity as one of the great reformers in tuberculin tests and as one who has done an immense amount of good to humanity. The skin test in twenty-four hours will show you whether the case is tubercular.... We should all of us as a society welcome Prof. von Pirquet. He is a foreigner whom we are proud to welcome.[3]

In a paper read before the Philadelphia Pediatric Society on February 8, 1910, von Pirquet discussed his cutaneous tuberculin test. Although the article contains many statements taken from previous communications, it is of interest for several reasons. First, it emphasized the disappointment which followed Koch's attempt at treating tuberculosis with tuberculin. Not until many years afterward was tuberculin, in far smaller doses, again generally applied in therapeutics. But one valuable lesson learned from the first period of tuberculization was its usefulness in diagnosis. Furthermore, the article is of interest because it contains a clear-cut, precise expression of the limitations of the test.

Von Pirquet believed that segregation of tuberculous and nontuberculous individuals could eradicate the disease, and he described his experience in making such a separation in a Baltimore orphanage for those of preschool age, where the entire population of 227 children was given the cutaneous test. In no instance was there a reaction in a child below one year of age; but positive

---

[3] C. von Pirquet, "The Relation of Tuberculosis to Infant Mortality," *New York Med. J.* 90 (1909): 1045.

reactions were obtained in six children whose ages were between one and three years, and in nineteen of those between four and six years of age. The older children who showed positive reactions were sent to the farm of the institution; the six smaller children were segregated in one room. In this way other young children who lived at the orphanage were prevented from contracting a tuberculous infection from their playmates. The only possibility of infection might arise from contact with members of the staff and they, of course, had to be carefully controlled. Such a separation would be worth while only in the first years of life and could only be carried out in an institution.

Von Pirquet noted that the cutaneous tuberculin reaction was merely one instance in which an infectious disease could be diagnosed on the basis of the antibody theory. The cutaneous test had already had practical application in the diagnosis of glanders of horses and the group of fungous infections caused by *Trichophyton* microorganisms, and was rapidly being developed.[4]

While in Baltimore he was invited to deliver the Annual Oration to the Faculty on April 27, 1910. He discussed medical teaching and stated in part: "The average student leaves our medical schools without having seen many of the infectious diseases of childhood. When entering on his practice, his ignorance contrasts sadly with the knowledge of mothers and grandmothers, gained by experience."

Some of von Pirquet's concepts have been replaced by new advances. We now have active immunization against diphtheria, whooping cough, poliomyelitis, and measles; and antibiotics are available for the treatment of scarlet fever. But even under present circumstances, when certain infectious diseases are so rare that the student has little opportunity to see a case during his course in pediatrics, he still needs the best possible training. In von Pirquet's time the infectious disease of childhood which produced the most serious consequences was tuberculosis. Not only has the incidence of tuberculous infection in childhood markedly decreased, but the disease has responded to treatment with drugs. Even tubercular meningitis, which had 100 per cent mortality, is now curable. In 1910 von Pirquet urged that "the medical student should get a good training in the ordinary in-

---

[4] "The Cutaneous Tuberculin Test," *Arch. Pediat.* 27 (1910): 161.

fectious diseases of childhood, in order to make the diagnosis with certainty, even in somewhat atypical cases, in order to apply the right therapy, to be able to make a prognosis, and in order to take prophylactic measures necessary for that individual case; finally, in order to distinguish a case of the dangerous, unusual infections which involve a real danger to the community." A theoretical course or an occasional case seen in a dispensary was not sufficient; he believed the students should be taught at the bedside by a teacher who himself had received thorough training in infectious diseases. He recommended that "wards for the common endemic infections should be attached to the hospitals of the medical schools. This from the hygienic standpoint is not only not objectionable but has many advantages. A certain number of hours of bedside instruction in infectious diseases should be inserted as a necessary course in the medical curriculum in the third or fourth year."[5]

His few other contributions during the Baltimore period—two chapters for a handbook of pediatrics, one on vaccination[6] and the other on serum sickness,[7] an article on allergy,[8] and a section on cutaneous tuberculin reactions for a technical handbook[9]— were but ramifications of previous work. The only original investigation consisted of quantitative experiments with the cutaneous tuberculin reaction. It, too, was related to previous studies, but he never continued the work. He talked about it occasionally, but never considered it one of his top achievements. The most striking feature—as in many of his papers—was the graphic analysis. He concluded that the cutaneous tuberculin reaction depended on at least two factors. One was the tuberculin; the other, furnished by the organism, could be considered as an antibody which originated during a previous infection with tubercle bacilli. In his experiments the first factor was subjected

[5] "The Importance of a Thorough Teaching of Infectious Diseases of Childhood in the Medical Curriculum," *Bull. Med.-Chir. Faculty of Maryland* (1910), 211.

[6] "Vakzination," in *Handbuch der Kinderheilkunde*, M. Pfaundler and A. Schlossmann, eds. (2d ed.; Leipzig: F. C. W. Vogel, 1910), 2: 247.

[7] C. von Pirquet, and B. Schick, "Serumkrankheit," in *Handbuch der Kinderheilkunde*, M. Pfaundler and A. Schlossmann, eds. (2d ed.; Leipzig: F. C. W. Vogel, 1910), 2: 584.

[8] "Allergy," *Arch. Int. Med.* 7 (1911): 259, 383.

[9] "Die lokalen Tuberkulinreaktionen," in *Handbuch der Technik und Methodik der Immunitätsforschung. I. Ergänzungsband* (Jena: Gustav Fischer, 1910), p. 191.

to definite variations by the use of different concentrations of tuberculin. The effect of progressive dilutions was to decrease the intensity of the reaction, as had occurred previously in the early reaction in cowpox vaccination. The effect could not be reduced to a definite mathematical expression, but von Pirquet postulated that the phenomena could be classed under the mass-action law. It was his impression "that the active mass of the second factor is very much smaller than the active mass of the tuberculin used in the reaction."

The presence of the second factor can only be surmised from the following considerations: An individual, free from any tubercular infection, does not give any cutaneous reactions with tuberculin. In persons who give the reaction, a marked difference exists between different areas of the skin. In skin areas which have been subjected previously to one or repeated applications of tuberculin, the reaction proceeds in a different manner. Here again a striking analogy with the results of repeated smallpox vaccinations becomes manifest, and it may be concluded that besides an accumulation of antibody in the general organism a local accumulation occurs. The inflammatory reaction is supposed to rest on a union of both the factors given, with the production of a toxic principle. This toxic principle acts on the tissues producing the inflammatory papules and reddened areas. A figure [p. 66 in *Important Medical Discoveries*] demonstrates the influence of the concentrations of tuberculin and supposed antibody on the course of the reaction.

. . . in every instance a period of latency was recorded, even when the high concentration of both factors induced a relatively rapid appearance of the reaction.[10]

Von Pirquet remained in Baltimore only about a year. In 1910 he took a leave of absence from The Johns Hopkins University, with the door open for a possible return.

March 6, 1910

Dear President Remsen,

Upon nomination by the Medical Faculty of the University of Breslau, the Prussian ministry of education has offered me the position of professor of Pediatrics at that University. I have accepted this call.

Mr. Blanchard Randall has suggested that I should not offer my resignation here, but that I should ask for a leave of absence and have a chance to consider the question again after having tried the position in Breslau. Mr. Randall's suggestion was very agreeable to me, as it gives

[10] "Quantitative Experiments with the Cutaneous Tuberculin Reaction," *J. Pharmacol. and Exper. Therap.* 1 (1909): 151.

me the possibility of coming back and continuing and developing the work here under more favorable conditions for both of us.

It would be gratifying to me if some such arrangement could be made by which my relations with the Johns Hopkins University and the Hospital were not completely severed at this time, so that I might assume the position in Breslau and still might have the opportunity, if on trial of this position it seemed to me best to return here, to be able to do so. Of course my salary would cease during my absence from the first of May and I should agree to communicate to you my final decision at least before the first of next January, it being understood that the University is at the same time free to fill my chair if it so desires. . . .

Three days later, Dr. Remsen sent the following reply:

Your communication of the 6th inst. was presented to our Board of Trustees at the meeting held on that date, and it was agreed to grant your request provided the Advisory Board of the Medical Faculty should so recommend. There can be no doubt that the Advisory Board will so recommend, and you may therefore take action accordingly.

Attempts were made to hold von Pirquet at Johns Hopkins. On January 31, 1911, the President of the Board of Trustees offered him the first full-time professorship in the history of The Johns Hopkins University. Surprisingly, the offer was made two years before the specialties of pediatrics, medicine, and surgery were formally established as full-time departments.

My dear Doctor,

On behalf of the Trustees of the Johns Hopkins University, I take pleasure in making you the following offer in connection with the professorship of Pediatrics:

A yearly salary of $7500 on condition that you devote yourself entirely to the care of hospital patients (both free and pay), teaching and investigation, and do not engage in private practice. You will have as complete control of the clinic as is possible under existing conditions. That is, you will have absolute control over the admission of a specified number of free patients, the power of veto in the choice of head nurses, a specified budget for laboratory and teaching purposes, a small petty cash account, and, through the Medical Board of the Hospital and the Faculty of the University, practically free choice of all your upper assistants. The general financial and economic administration of the department will, however, remain in the hands of the Hospital Trustees.

Such a position will make you eligible for a Carnegie pension, which would provide for you and your wife after retirement.

In order to make possible the payment of so large a salary, which will be the largest thus far paid to any professor in the University, you and your assistants will be expected to supervise the treatment of all private patients admitted to the Children's Hospital with the understanding that whatever fees are paid for such service will go into the Treasury of the Hospital and not to you.

Naturally, the pecuniary returns from such an arrangement may be much less than if you engaged in private or consulting practice, but, on the other hand, there will be certain compensations, such as uninterrupted time for work, greater facility for investigation, a regular income and finally a retiring pension.

We hope that arrangements may ultimately be made which will enable us to put the heads of the other main departments of the Hospital upon a similar basis. If this is done, the maximum salary will probably be $10,000 a year, in which you would naturally share. Even if such an arrangement does not prove feasible, we should look forward to advancing your salary to that figure, whenever the fees from pay patients in your department become sufficiently large to justify the expenditure.

Hoping that the proposition will be acceptable to you, and looking forward to having you with us next year.

P.S. Patients may be seen outside of the Hospital in consultation with physicians in cases of scientific interest or urgent necessity. The fees, however, will go to the Hospital, as otherwise the right to a Carnegie pension would be vitiated.

Even after von Pirquet was invited to go to the University of Vienna the junior members of the faculty of the Medical Department of The Johns Hopkins University sent a memorandum to the president, signed by forty-one members, together with a subscription toward any fund necessary for his salary. This important document shows the high esteem in which von Pirquet was held by his colleagues:

Baltimore, April 27, 1911

Whereas, we have learned with pride that the Directorship of the Imperial Pediatric Clinic of the University of Vienna has been tendered to a member of the Faculty of the Johns Hopkins University, Professor Clemens von Pirquet; and whereas, by virtue of this offer as well as the brilliancy of his researches he is officially recognized as one of the foremost living pediatricians; and whereas, during his stay in Baltimore Professor von Pirquet has by precept and example become a source of exceptional personal inspiration to us all.

We, the undersigned junior members of the Faculty of the Medical Department of the Johns Hopkins University, respectfully beg to express our deep appreciation of the services of Professor von Pirquet to the Johns Hopkins Medical School, as well as to medical education in America in general, and to express the hope that these services may not be lost to the University; and in accordance with this sentiment we do hereby subscribe $2500.00 toward any fund necessary for his salary during the next year in Baltimore.

The offer was not accepted, and on May 2 the president directed a reply to Dr. Samuel Amberg and others.

Gentlemen:

Through the Dean of the Medical Faculty the resolutions adopted by certain junior members of the Faculty of the Medical Department of the Johns Hopkins University, have come into my hands.

At the regular meeting of the Board of Trustees of the Johns Hopkins University held May 1, I read these resolutions. The Trustees were much gratified by your action and especially pleased by the spirit shown by you. Let me assure you that everything reasonable that can be done to secure the return of Dr. von Pirquet will be done. The Trustees fully appreciate the value of his services and the offer which has been made by me is such that it does not seem probable that he will decline for financial reasons, whatever he may do for other reasons. We are now awaiting his reply.

While the Trustees appreciate your generosity and self sacrifice in making the offer you have made, they do not feel that they should accept your subscription under the circumstances.

Meanwhile, on May 1, President Remsen had sent the following letter:

Dear Professor von Pirquet:

On the thirty-first of January I wrote you a letter making an offer of the professorship of pediatrics in this University. A copy of that letter was sent to you on March second, as no answer had been received up to that time.

It is now necessary that we should have your reply, for which we have waited as long as possible in the hope that you could see your way clear to accept.

The Trustees at their last meeting requested me to communicate with you and secure your answer. Will you kindly cable me your reply soon after receipt of this letter.

Von Pirquet's reply bore the date line of Breslau, June 27, 1911:

DEAR PRESIDENT REMSEN,

I am in receipt of your letter of January the 31st, and a copy of it sent on March 2nd, and finally of a letter of May 1st. I cabled twice in reply of the last one.

The reason why I did not answer your first letter was that I wanted to communicate with Mr. Randall and some of the professors about several points of the offer, before giving you an official and definite reply.

The main point was that, although I was very much in favor of devoting myself entirely to the care of hospital patients, teaching and investigation, I did not consider a yearly salary of $7500 an adequate remuneration under these circumstances. I stated that for a salary of $10,000 I would be willing to accept your offer.

Meantime I have learned from Mr. Randall that you were not able to pay this sum and that you did not consider favorably the idea of the Johns Hopkins Alumni to contribute toward the amount asked for. Under the circumstances, to my great regret, I must decline your invitation, as I cabled you in my recent telegram.

I have accepted the offer of the Imperial University of Vienna to be the successor of my teacher Prof. Escherich.

Let me thank you on this occasion once more for the many kindnesses which you showed me during my stay in Baltimore. I may assure you that in the future I shall always keep in memory the pleasure of having worked with the Johns Hopkins faculty and of having been in association with such a fine body of students.

Please remember me to the Trustees and the Faculty.

Escherich's tragic death on February 15 during a lecture to his students, and the opportunity for von Pirquet to return to his native country, obviously made the decision very easy. In the autumn of 1911 he assumed the chair of pediatrics at the University of Vienna, where he remained until the end of his life.

VII

Breslau

In 1910, von Pirquet became professor of pediatrics at the University of Breslau, then in Germany.[1] By a decree of the academic senate of the university on June 11, he was at the same time appointed an o.ö. (ordinary public) professor and director of the University Children's Hospital. He held these positions throughout two summer terms and the intervening winter session, until October 1, 1911.

We know little of his private life in Breslau. Rowntree, who went to see the von Pirquets there in 1910, commented on his visit in a chapter headed "There Were Giants in Europe in Those Days":

> In the early years of this century, the most famous child specialist of Europe was Dr. von Pirquet. His interests were broad. He was a leader in the development of pediatrics, of infant feeding, and studies in sensitivities of all kinds. . . .
>
> On arriving at Breslau I phoned Dr. von Pirquet. He came over to see us and invited us to his home for dinner. My sister and Mrs. von Pirquet formed quite an attachment. Mrs. von Pirquet . . . was a very charming but an unusual and rather strange woman. She smoked excessively, even at that early date.[2]

Some information about this period was provided by Franz von Gröer,[3] a native of Warsaw (then in the Russian part of Poland), who worked on his doctoral thesis in Breslau and attended von Pirquet's lectures. They met first socially and von Gröer was pleased and impressed that he, an unknown student, should be treated with such cordiality by the Professor of Pediatrics. Von Pirquet gave him a letter of recommendation to a leading bacteriologist in St. Petersburg to help him obtain the necessary credit

[1] When Breslau was ceded to Poland, it was renamed Wroclaw.

[2] L. G. Rowntree, *Amid Masters of Twentieth Century Medicine* (Springfield, Illinois: C. C Thomas, 1958). (Courtesy of Charles C Thomas, publisher, Springfield.)

[3] Personal communication.

for the Russian doctor's degree. Von Gröer was stimulated by von Pirquet's lectures to enter the field of pediatrics. Later he followed von Pirquet to Vienna and held an appointment at the *Kinderklinik* until he himself became professor of pediatrics at Lwów, Poland. Von Pirquet was generally held in high regard and many other students were similarly impressed. The women were particularly attracted by his personality, and there were rumors of Madame von Pirquet's jealousy.

Von Pirquet's scientific accomplishments in Breslau indicate rather concentrated activity for a period of sixteen months, especially since they were performed in addition to his student lectures and the examinations. At a Breslau medical meeting he introduced himself to his new medical confreres and gave a succinct discussion of his concept of allergy. He stated that, in theory, the ability of an organism to react may be altered by the effects of disease or by prophylactic treatment with bacterial products or other foreign substances. This alteration may be (1) a *temporary* change in the speed of reaction, either immediate or accelerated; (2) a *quantitative* change in which the reaction is either increased (hypersensitivity, anaphylaxis), diminished, or abolished (reduced sensitivity or immunity); or (3) a *qualitative* change in reaction and in the reacting tissue. Passive anaphylaxis from injection of serum containing the antibody and antianaphylaxis, and neutralization of the antibody by previously injected antigen, are other possibilities.

Up to that time biologists had been interested chiefly in the constitutional symptoms resulting from a second injection which produced death in experimental animals. Such basic symptoms depended upon the formation of apotoxin, the toxic complex resulting from the reaction of antigen and antibody. Von Pirquet stated that the more obscure clinical findings presumably depended upon whether more apotoxin was produced in the nervous system, on the skin, or in the lung.

After intravenous injection the mode of fixation, and hence the target of the toxins, differs with individuals and species. In his experiments, von Pirquet preferred cutaneous or subcutaneous injection so that the apotoxin could be clearly observed on the surface of the skin. He likened this procedure to selection of a peripheral point for studying the effect of electric current on an experimental animal. Intravenous injection was comparable to passing the current through the entire body and observing the death of the animal instead of a twitching.[4]

Another article written in Breslau, described as the double reaction at the cowpox vaccination, referred to an analogous phenomenon in serum sickness. Von Pirquet recapitulated his previous observations of immediate and accelerated reactions (Fig. 13). In addition, a third category included cases showing both reactions in sequence, or *double reaction*. Although the double reaction can occur at any time, it usually appears after an interval of one to six months[5] (Fig. 14).

The experiences with serum sickness had been relatively simple. In cowpox vaccination, on the other hand, an additional factor— the development of the vaccinial organism in the skin—seemed at first to obscure the reactions between foreign protein and antibody. Von Pirquet showed that, after injection of heat-killed cowpox vaccine, subcutaneous reactions appeared in previously vaccinated individuals. They resembled both the specific edema described by von Pirquet and Schick after reinjection with foreign serum and the puncture reaction of Escherich in tuberculous individuals. However, the vaccinial puncture reaction differed from the other two in that it did not show the urticaria-like character of the skin, the intensive itching of the specific-serum edema, the dark discoloration, or the pain on pressure of the subcutaneous tuberculin reaction. It was characterized by a reddish-yellow discoloration and was completely painless. The incubation time with heat-killed cowpox vaccine was not always twenty-four to forty-eight hours, but an "accelerated reaction" of several days might be exhibited.

When cutaneous vaccination was carried out with fresh cowpox vaccine, previously vaccinated individuals might show either an immediate apotoxic reaction or an accelerated reaction.[6] In the latter case the vaccinia virus caused formation of a colony in the skin, as with a first vaccination, and vanished in an accelerated manner. Figure 13 shows the differences between immediate, accelerated, and normal reaction time in vaccination. In this

---

[4] "Medizinische Sektion der schlesischen Gesellschaft für vaterländische Kultur zu Breslau," *Berlin. klin. Wchnschr.* 47, no. 51 (1910).

[5] "Die Doppelreaktion bei der Kuhpockenimpfung," *München. med. Wchnschr.* 58 (1911): 937.

[6] Described in detail by von Pirquet in his monograph, *Klinische Studien über Vaccination und vaccinale Allergie* (Vienna: Franz Deuticke, 1907), pp. 84–107.

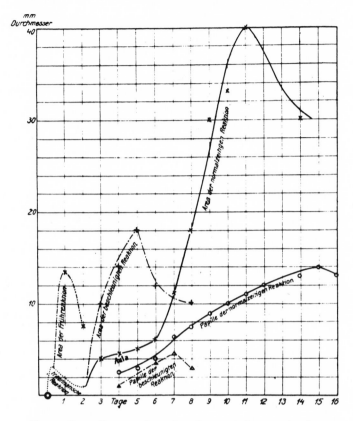

Fig. 13. Immediate, accelerated, and normal time reaction in cow-pox vaccination.

Traumatische Reaktion—traumatic reaction
Area der Frühreaktion—area of early reaction
Area der beschleunigten Reaktion—area of accelerated reaction
Area der normalzeitigen Reaktion—area of normal time reaction
Papille der beschleunigten Reaktion—papilla of accelerated reaction
Papille der normalzeitigen Reaktion—papilla of normal time reaction
(Vertical scale—Diameter [mm.].) *From:* "Die Doppelreaktion bei der Kuhpockenimpfung," *München. med. Wchnschr.* 58 (1911): 937. (Courtesy of J. F. Lehmanns Verlag, Munich.)

experiment immediate and accelerated reactions did not take place at the same vaccination or injection. However, there were also cases where—in analogy with the double reaction following serum administration—immediate and accelerated reactions appeared successively following revaccination. On simultaneous revaccination and injection with heat-killed vaccine, four years after the primary vaccination, an early reaction first developed

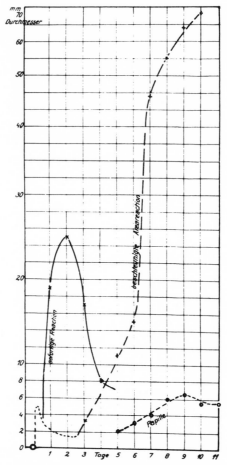

Fig. 14. Double reaction in cowpox vaccination. The solid line shows the extension of immediate reaction at the site of injection; the interrupted line, the course of accelerated area reaction. Growth of the papilla was stopped at the time of maximum development.

Sofortige Reaktion—immediate reaction

Beschleunigte Areareaktion—accelerated area reaction

Papille—papilla

(Vertical scale—Diameter [mm.].) *From:* "Die Doppelreaktion bei der Kuhpockenimpfung," *München. med. Wchnschr.* 58 (1911): 937. (Courtesy of J. F. Lehmanns Verlag, Munich.)

at the site of the injection, attaining its maximum after forty-eight hours, and thereafter an accelerated reaction appeared at one of the sites of cutaneous vaccination.

In another case von Pirquet observed both the primary vaccination with its normal reaction time and the double reaction, 112 days later. The primary vaccination on July 25, 1910, had all the characteristics of a primary take. On November 4, after 102 days, a cutaneous vaccination with fresh cowpox vaccine was given at two spots, as well as an injection of 0.1 cc. of a 10 per cent heated vaccine. There was no detectable reaction. Six days later the same experiment resulted in a trace of reaction at the site of the vaccination and a small puncture reaction at the site of the injection. On November 14 the experiment was repeated with the variation that 0.1 cc. of an unheated, undiluted vaccine was cutaneously injected instead of the heated 10 per cent vaccine. First an early reaction appeared at the site of the injection and an area of redness 18 by 15 mm.; in the center was an itchy papule which decreased the next day. Second, an accelerated reaction developed at the site of the injection and also at one of the points of vaccination. At the site of the vaccination the following change could be observed: four days after vaccination the reddening was 25 mm. in diameter, increasing to 38 mm. in six days. A small vesicle in the center attained a diameter of 5 mm. and finally became encrusted. On December 6 (134 days after vaccination) four vaccinations and one injection with diluted vaccine were carried out. At all points an early reaction occurred. The findings were the same when the experiment was repeated on February 24, 1911 (214 days following the primary vaccination).

It is striking that a cluster formed at the site so soon after the first vaccination. Von Pirquet attributed this absence of immunity to the simultaneous injection of unchanged vaccine, suggesting that the latter deprived the organism of "ergines" to such an extent that attenuation of all pathogens could no longer be attained.

The relation of hypersensitivity and immunity to cowpox vaccination cast a sidelight on the insensitiveness toward tuberculin and its relation to resistance toward the injection with tubercle bacilli. From these experiments he drew the following conclusions:

1. As in serum sickness, an immediate, an accelerated, and a double allergic reaction can be distinguished in cowpox vaccination.
2. The accelerated reaction can be observed after cutaneous inoculation of virulent vaccine as well as after subcutaneous injection of heat-killed vaccine.

A few other articles and textbook contributions were written

during this period. The classic textbook of pediatrics at that time
for students in the German-speaking countries was that of Feer,[7]
a work comparable to Nelson's textbook in this country. Because
chapters were contributed by outstanding specialists in the field
of pediatrics, the book had a wide circulation and not until after
Feer's death was it supplanted. Von Pirquet's chapters dealt with
diseases of the respiratory organs and with tuberculosis. No one
but he had the necessary experience and competence in these
subjects. Even after more than fifty years the chapter on tuberculosis is still a classic, although it was written before the development of X-ray diagnosis. Except for addition of that subject, no
essential change was required in subsequent editions.

A lecture on tuberculosis in childhood, delivered on February
10, 1911, is significant only because it showed von Pirquet's
unfavorable attitude toward treatment with tuberculin, which
at that time was having a short period of popularity in Germany.[8]
A comprehensive article, which appeared the same year, on the
types of allergic reaction found at revaccination set forth chiefly
the highlights of previous studies and described the clinical effects:
accelerated reaction with and without formation of a papilla,
torpid papule reaction, early reaction, double reaction (early and
accelerated at the place of vaccination), and keloid formation.
The different types were explained by the behavior of the vaccinial colony and by the antibodies, whether they were already
present or formed by accelerated reproduction. Hypersensitivity
(the result of an intracutaneous reaction toward heat-killed
vaccine) and immunity (measured by the number of sites of
vaccination cut off in their development) were said to be closely
associated in the vaccinial allergy.[9]

Even though von Pirquet's accomplishments at the University
of Breslau were significant, he soon realized that he had not made
a happy choice. His position produced many demands of an
administrative nature which interfered with his research interests.
Neither was stimulation to be found in the city itself, which from
its border position in Silesia had long been a political football.
Consequently it lacked the traditional and cultural charm usually

---

[7] E. Feer, *Lehrbuch der Kinderheilkunde* (Jena: Gustav Fischer, 1911).
[8] "Ueber Tuberkulose des Kindesalters," *Berlin. klin. Wchnschr.* 48 (1911): 595.
[9] "Ueber die verschiedenen Formen der allergischen Reaktion bei der Revaccination," *Ztschr. f. Immunitätsforschung u. exper. Therap.* 10 (1911): 1.

found in the environs of a distinguished university. Von Pirquet was still on leave of absence from The Johns Hopkins University and was considering a return to Baltimore when Escherich died unexpectedly. The invitation to succeed his renowned teacher at the University of Vienna came soon thereafter and was accepted gladly.

VIII

Vienna

Pediatrics had followed a distinguished course in Vienna for a century before von Pirquet became professor there. Its development was traced by Max Neuburger, medical historian, and his original article, translated by Robert Rosenthal, forms the basis for this historical outline.

Before the advent of pediatrics the sick child was usually cared for by a midwife, wet nurse, or elderly woman rather than by a physician. This choice reflected both a popular lack of confidence in medical treatment and the physician's own reluctance to deal with patients unable to describe their complaints. Medicine still lacked the objective physical diagnosis. Pediatrics became a medical specialty in Vienna toward the end of the eighteenth century. It was advanced not by institutions connected with a university but by those established from a humanitarian viewpoint, which were encouraged during the era of Emperor Joseph. In 1784 the *Allgemeines Krankenhaus* was founded, and at the same time the first orphanage was built in Vienna. The abundance of pediatric cases induced physicians to devote increasing time and attention to this field.

Vienna's *Kinderkrankeninstitut*, founded by Joseph Johann Mastalier, gave free medical treatment to children from 1787 until 1938, either at the dispensary or in their homes. After Mastalier's death the dispensary became a public institution, and Leopold Anton Gölis served as its director for thirty-three years. Under his successful management the services were expanded and an affiliated vaccination institute was established. During the first twenty-five years of his tenure more than 130,000 infants and children were examined in the dispensary and over 10,000 were vaccinated. For his far-reaching, scientific work Gölis was justly called the founder of pediatrics in Austria.

In 1837 Dr. Ludwig Wilhelm Mauthner opened at his own expense a twelve-bed children's hospital and dispensary in the populous suburb of Schottenfeld. This institution was the first of its kind in Austria. Europe then had two others—the *Hôpital des enfants malades* in Paris (1802) and the Nicolai Children's Hospital in St. Petersburg (1834). Mauthner's dispensary clinic was extremely popular and physicians from Austria and from abroad went there to study. The high quality of teaching is shown by Neuburger's statement: "Pathological anatomical dissections were carefully carried out and interesting specimens were given to the Josephinian Academy for safekeeping after drawings had been made by artists who attended the autopsy." Later Mauthner obtained permission to present patients at his lectures. He also established a school for training pediatric nurses. The hospital was taken over by a benevolent society, moved to a suburb, and named the St. Anna Children's Hospital. Mauthner's clinic became a teaching institute of the university, and in 1851 he was named extraordinary professor of pediatrics.

Following Mauthner's death in 1858, he was succeeded by Franz Mayer, whose "didactic and literary work fitted splendidly into the frame of the Vienna school." Mayer, formerly assistant physician and superintendent of the St. Joseph Children's Hospital, did particularly good work in symptomatology and the description of diseases.

After St. Joseph's was built in 1842 the *Kronprinz Rudolph* and the Karolinen hospitals soon followed. Their staff physicians were active in practice and in research. This dynamic scientific life, shown by the increase in pediatric publications, resulted in controversies which occasionally led to sharp attacks. "It remained for Hermann Widerhofer, the successor of Mayer, and third director of the Vienna Pediatric Clinic, to bring about a peaceful settlement." He was an inspiration to others, and under his guidance the Vienna School became the center of German pediatrics. For almost forty years Widerhofer taught medical students and the many physicians who were attracted by the extensive clinical material and the stimulating method of teaching, so well suited to the needs of the practicing pediatrician.

In 1859 he became extraordinary professor of pediatrics; twenty-five years later he was made ordinary professor, the first to hold the chair of pediatrics at the University of Vienna. Widerhofer's strength lay in centering the physical examination on the immediate problem, in prompt recognition of the findings pertinent to diagnosis, and in his capacity to present a well-rounded clinical picture. He emphasized good diet and hygiene, with a minimum of complicated medications. His thinking and his explanations were clear and his publications, although few, are of permanent value. An essay on diseases of the bronchial glands, based on profound anatomical research, shows that Widerhofer was the first to understand the importance of the tuberculous involvement of these glands.

Escherich was invited to become professor of pediatrics in Vienna after Widerhofer's death in 1902. For twelve years he had been chief of the children's clinic in Graz, where he founded a school which became well known, carried out research, and was a very successful organizer. He, Heubner, and Czerny were the undisputed leaders in German pediatrics. Escherich believed in preventive pediatrics as well as in research and cure; and was interested in every phase of the specialty. He published almost two hundred articles. His bacteriological studies included a classical work on the intestinal flora of infants; discovery of the *Bacterium coli commune*, which has come to be known as *Escherichia coli*, and of the colicystitis and enteritis of infants caused by streptococci; work on diphtheria, on the parathyroid etiology of tetany, on infant feeding and digestion, and on the *Stichreaktion* of tuberculosis with which his name is associated.

Escherich was an excellent teacher who encouraged his assistants in their scientific investigations. He modernized and remodeled the St. Anna Children's Hospital, built laboratories, a model infant department, and a school to train pediatric nurses. He founded a society for infant welfare; he was active in introducing physicians into the schools; he helped to organize child research in which physicians and educators could co-operate, a state institute for care of mothers and infants, and a Vienna pediatric society for the exchange of scientific ideas.[1] A new *Kinderklinik* was built according to Escherich's plans but he died suddenly in 1911, as the institution was being completed.

Two other historical works provide additional data about von Pirquet. Professor Erna Lesky, director of the Institute for the History of Medicine in Vienna, prepared an excellent two-page biographical sketch in which she presented the outstanding

[1] Max Neuburger, "Zur Geschichte der Wiener Kinderheilkunde," *Wien. med. Wchnschr.* 85 (1935): 197. Translation by Robert Rosenthal. "The History of Pediatrics in Vienna," *Med. Rec.* 156 (1943): 746.

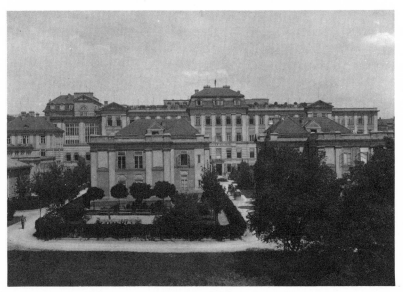

The *Kinderklinik.*

aspects of his work;[2] and Leopold Schoenbauer, in his book on medicine in Vienna, emphasized the significance of von Pirquet's contributions to pediatrics and science.[3]

Von Pirquet was keenly aware of the importance of preserving the tradition of fine pediatric teaching for which Vienna was justly famous, and he was successful in carrying on and even surpassing the ideals of his predecessors. The attitude toward medical education which he manifested in the annual oration to the faculty at The Johns Hopkins Medical School in 1910 was emphasized during his subsequent years in Vienna. His first lecture to the students after he became head of the Department of Pediatrics dealt with the nature of their education. The opening lecture of the newly appointed professor, on November 13, 1911, coincided with the dedication of the *Kinderklinik.* To this formal gathering, members of the Ministry of Education, civil service officials, faculty, and other guests had been invited. The occasion was made solemn by the recent death of Escherich, for whom one pavilion was to have been named.

[2] Erna Lesky, "Clemens von Pirquet," *Wien. klin. Wchnschr.* 67 (1955): 638.
[3] Leopold Schoenbauer, *Das Medizinische Wien* (Berlin: Urban and Schwarzenberg, 1947), pp. 359–61.

In the opening lecture von Pirquet dealt with the *Kinderklinik* as a hospital and as a teaching and research institution. He believed that the instruction of medical students should be predominantly practical, that students should learn how to deal with patients, and that they should implant live images upon their memories by seeing and examining as many patients as possible. He stressed again, as he had in Baltimore, the need for the physician to recognize readily the infectious diseases of childhood. No prophylaxis existed for the many cases of diphtheria and whooping cough, and only prompt treatment could avoid disastrous consequences for the child. Von Pirquet also realized that nothing could so damage a young physician's professional reputation as to be outdone in diagnosis by a grandmother.[4]

As the teaching progressed a full academic term was devoted to the contagious diseases and medical problems of childhood. This did not include infants, who were studied during the summer term, when nutritional disorders were rampant among those being fed cow's milk. Laboratory tests and microscopic techniques were not emphasized because they were a part of the student's prior education which he was expected to remember and draw upon.

By always keeping in mind when making ward rounds that beside him was an individual student whose knowledge was representative of that of his colleagues, von Pirquet avoided theoretical discussions which might be above or below the student level. For the same reason he limited instruction in infant nutrition to a few well-established basic principles, without much detail. Emphasis was placed on physical examination and on treatment of such common conditions as nutritional disorders, bronchitis, rickets, and constipation, which are often overlooked in medical education.

Three mornings a week von Pirquet presided at student lectures, with case presentation, in the amphitheater. He was one of the first to realize that, although physicians of his own and of previous generations had been trained in the art of medicine, the early twentieth century was a period of transition from art to science. Discoveries were being made so rapidly that one man's knowledge could no longer encompass all branches of medicine. Each of the assistants in the *Kinderklinik* was trained in one of the pediatric

[4] "Die neue Kinderklinik als Heil-, Lehr- und Forschungsinstitut," *Wien. med. Wchnschr.* 61 (1911): 2998.

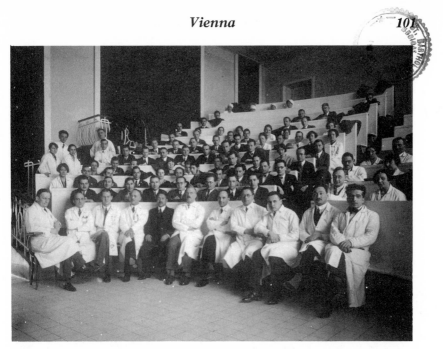

Staff and undergraduate students in amphitheater. Von Pirquet is seated in front row. At his right, in business suit, is a visiting Japanese physician; at his left, the author.

subspecialties—hematology, metabolism and endocrinology, neurology, psychiatry—and when a suitable case was presented von Pirquet would step from the platform while an assistant discussed a problem which concerned his subspecialization. Although radiology was not yet a pediatric subspecialty, at the *Kinderklinik* the radiologist was required to be a trained pediatrician.

The postgraduate seminars which the University of Vienna offered to practicing physicians included a lecture by von Pirquet and one by each of his seven assistants. Copies of each lecture were printed and distributed in advance to enable the participants to take part in the discussion. On one occasion von Pirquet had procrastinated in preparing his lecture. As the date approached, the chairman for the postgraduate teaching program sent a reminder. Still nothing was written, and a few days in advance a telephone call was received. Von Pirquet referred the call to me and I told the chairman that I would be responsible for preparing the lecture material and sending it to him. As I finished the conversation, von Pirquet quoted La Fontaine: "And so the obstinate donkey got rid of the hated burden."

Another responsibility which had become burdensome to him was the revision of three chapters which appeared in Feer's textbook. Von Pirquet wrote his chapters in 1910, but rapid advances required that they be brought up to date annually for each revision of the book. By the time I became associated with him in 1919 he was thoroughly tired of working over the same material and checking the proofs. He was delighted to relinquish the task, and as he turned the material over to me he said, "It gives me indigestion."

The mothers always brought a large number of acutely ill children to the hospital in the morning, and for many years it was my privilege to select from the wards and outpatient department the cases for discussion and to estimate how many would be needed for the two-hour lecture. At the end of the session von Pirquet would call for the clinic patients who had come for the first time. He took a history in the presence of the students by questioning the child's parent or grandparent, and made a tentative diagnosis. A seriously ill child would be admitted to the hospital; otherwise the patient was asked to return for follow-up. His teaching was always stimulating and, as in Breslau, students and physicians came to von Pirquet's *Klinik*—as the Pediatric Department became known—for specialty training.

During the years that he was director of the *Kinderklinik*, von Pirquet's career was one of striking contrasts. His work displayed brilliant productivity and failing powers, scientific advances acclaimed by the world yet rejected by his profession, dedication to saving the lives of others culminated by destruction of his own life. Management of the patients and of student teaching was well organized and the duties were shared with several assistants, so that, even in the later years when his interests lay elsewhere, the *Kinderklinik* maintained its worldwide renown.

While in Vienna von Pirquet produced a highly original theory of the skin rash in measles which was related to his early work on allergy. This penetrating study is a masterpiece of graphic analysis and a fine example of his way of thinking. After first devising the theory, he proceeded to verify it by making precise recordings of the skin rash on forty-six patients with measles. Initially he photographed the eruption, but found that the appearance on successive days could be presented more satisfactorily by means of drawings (Fig. 15). In ten patients he studied the earliest signs of the rash, depicting its course during the first day. In nine others the subsequent course and the fading of the rash were observed, and drawings were made of its appearance from the second to the fifth day.

In all of the patients, local factors exerted a strong influence. The rash appeared earlier on hyperemic areas, such as those

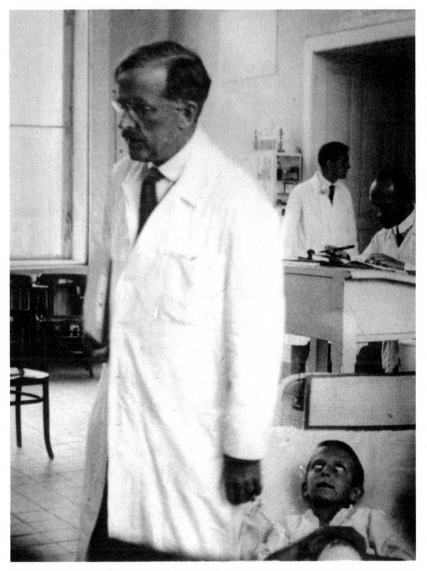

Von Pirquet and the author (at desk) in the lecture hall.

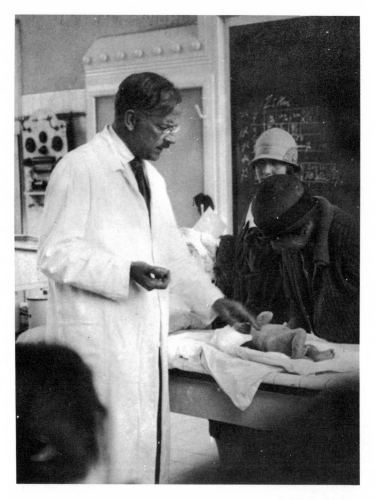

Von Pirquet in the lecture hall with infant and grandmother.

produced by a positive tuberculin test, the pressure of garters, or chafing, than on normal skin. When erythema multiforme or urticaria had occurred previously the pattern of measles was almost completely reversed in that the rash appeared first on the extremities, which usually did not become involved until after the trunk. It was dense on the skin surrounding a scar, scanty on the scar itself. Several experiments showed that the eruption was encouraged by artificial stimulation of the skin or passive congestion applied at least one day before the appearance of the rash.

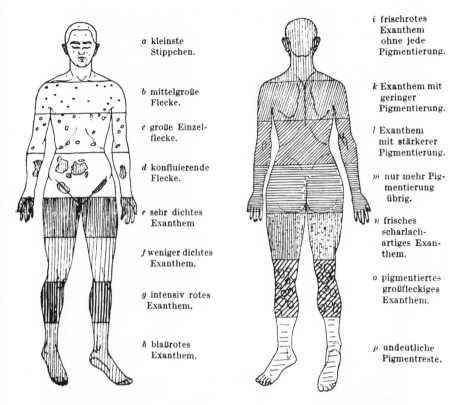

a kleinste
Stippchen.

b mittelgroße
Flecke.

c große Einzel-
flecke.

d konfluierende
Flecke.

e sehr dichtes
Exanthem

f weniger dichtes
Exanthem.

g intensiv rotes
Exanthem.

h blaßrotes
Exanthem.

i frischrotes
Exanthem
ohne jede
Pigmentierung.

k Exanthem mit
geringer
Pigmentierung.

l Exanthem
mit stärkerer
Pigmentierung.

m nur mehr Pig-
mentierung
übrig.

n frisches
scharlach-
artiges Exan-
them.

o pigmentiertes
großfleckiges
Exanthem.

p undeutliche
Pigmentreste.

Fig. 15. Sketch of the skin rash in measles.

a. Smallest specks
b. Medium-sized spots
c. Large single spots
d. Confluent spots
e. Very dense exanthem
f. Less dense exanthem
g. Deep red exanthem
h. Pale red exanthem

i. Emerging red exanthem with no
pigmentation
k. Exanthem with slight pigmentation
l. Exanthem with more pigmentation
m. Remnants of pigmentation
n. Emergent scarlatiniform exanthem
o. Pigmented exanthem consisting of
large spots
p. Indistinct remnants of pigment

From: *Das Bild der Masern auf der äusseren Haut* (Berlin: Julius Springer, 1913). (Courtesy of Springer–Verlag, Heidelberg.)

Its distribution did not follow the zones of Head and hence was unrelated to the pattern of sensory nerves. On the other hand, similarities could be demonstrated with the course of arteries. For the most part the rash erupted first on sites nearest the heart and the great vessels and in the presence of active circulation. It erupted later as the distance from the heart increased, as the blood had to travel a longer distance through small vessels, and with decreasing hyperemia of the site.

The observed facts and comparisons with findings in variola and vaccinia suggested to von Pirquet that the exanthema resulted from apotoxic reactions to measles organisms which had settled in the capillaries of the skin. His hypothesis states that the organisms causing measles become agglutinated as they pass through the capillaries of a skin area which is saturated with antibodies. Saturation of the surface of the skin is consequently the precipitating cause and precondition for the rash. Saturation is envisaged as taking place in much the same way that oxygen is delivered from the arterial blood. Thus the descent of the rash can be explained, those areas being saturated first which either show a very intensive circulation (mucous membranes) or are situated near the heart or the large blood vessels. Thereafter, other areas gradually receive sufficient amounts of antibodies to cause agglutination of the measles virus. By the agglutination, the causative organism is gradually filtered out from the circulation. At the ends of the extremities, which are saturated last, only a few antibodies remain available for agglutination, and there the rash is scanty and transient. It is frequently absent from elbows, feet, and buttocks because no more organisms are present in the blood stream at a time when the areas of poorest arterialization become saturated with antibodies.[5]

Even though the theory was never proved beyond a doubt, no other interpretation for the eruption of a rash has been offered. The theory may well be applied to other conditions in which an antigen-antibody reaction is to be expected and should be classed as one of von Pirquet's more significant contributions.

Another significant observation, made at about the same time, was an adjunct to the classical study of vaccination and vaccinial allergy of his early period. He distinguished the usual reaction to vaccination from a manifestation which he called *paravaccine*. After vaccination the expected sequence is that a small papule will form at the site of inoculation which becomes a vesicle, is pustular, surrounded by a red areola, and forms a crust which falls off to leave a white scar. Paravaccine, on the other hand, has a small, strictly circumscribed area of mild infection which is slower to develop, produces no itching or systemic manifestations,

[5] *Das Bild der Masern auf der äusseren Haut* (Berlin: Julius Springer, 1913).

and is characterized by a cherry-red color. It heals like a flat wart and leaves no scar. After revaccination the physician may have difficulty in differentiating the allergic signs of vaccinia from paravaccine. The presence of even a tiny scar indicates a vaccinia, as does termination of the reaction within a week. A slow course, of perhaps three weeks' duration, favors paravaccine. When doubt exists, the vaccination should be repeated.

Paravaccine is observed most frequently after inoculation with attenuated virus and a weak scarification of the skin. The reaction reaches a diameter of 4 to 6 mm. in the second week. Its occurrence after both primary and repeated vaccinations indicates that it is not an allergic modification of the vaccinia. It can be transmitted to the same or to another individual and retains the characteristics which distinguish it from vaccinia. It does not confer either immunity or allergy toward subsequent infection with vaccinia and is of significance only as it may simulate and mask true vaccinial effects.[6]

The paravaccine is apparently produced by specific organisms contained in the vaccine of calves, and has been reported in various countries. In France, for instance, it is known as *vaccine rouge*. Had it occurred in the early days when vaccination was carried out by direct transmission from one human to another, the sharp-eyed old observers would have described it as a conspicuous modification of vaccination.

As mentioned earlier, von Pirquet was of an inventive nature; one of his ideas was put into practice on the infants' ward of the *Kinderklinik*. The customary practice was to isolate all patients with nonairborne infections and diagnostic problems by placing them in enclosed chambers having glass sides and top and supplied with an exhaust and ventilating system. The chambers required a great deal of space and von Pirquet wanted a method of isolating infants, particularly those with respiratory infections, within the infant's ward itself. At first he experimented with a single crib in which the railings were replaced by glass; one side could be lowered like a sash window. This he called an isolation bed. Later, six such beds of two different sizes were assembled into a compact unit, thus reducing by one-third the number of glass walls. The walls were high enough to prevent the spread of droplet infection from coughing or sneezing. This block of six isola-

[6] "Die Paravaccine," *Ztschr. f. Kinderheilk.* 23 (1915): 309.

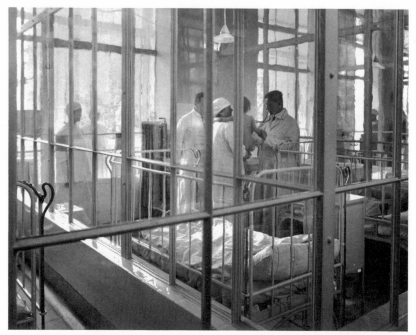

Ward with cubicles for isolation of patients with nonairborne infections.

tion beds occupied no more space in the ward than had formerly
been needed to accommodate three separated cribs. A small
cabinet to hold utensils for each infant was attached to the outside.
Adequate natural ventilation was afforded by the open top and
by an open space of several centimeters surrounding the mattress.
The temperature within the enclosures was the same as in the
rest of the ward.

The isolation beds proved satisfactory in protecting premature
infants and the newborn from those suffering from respiratory
infections and from staff or visitors who might be carrying such
infection. They did not, of course, afford protection against such
airborne infections as measles or chickenpox.[7]

Von Pirquet also objected to the common practice of placing
all newborn infants in one nursery and carrying them to the
mothers only for feeding. He believed that a baby should remain
with its mother in order to arouse her maternal instinct—the
concept of "rooming-in" which child psychiatrists have redis-
covered and now recommend.

[7] "Isolierbetten," *Ztschr. f. d. ges. Krankenhaus.* 24 (1928): 741.

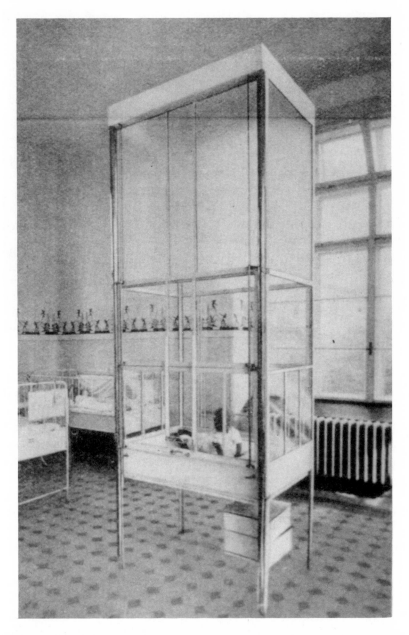

Isolation bed devised by von Pirquet. Although shown separately here, six such beds were assembled into a space-saving unit. *From:* "Isolierbetten," *Ztschr. f. d. ges. Krankenhauswesen* 24 (1928): 741. (Courtesy of Springer–Verlag, Heidelberg.)

Children who were admitted to the *Kinderklinik* for any problem were first given a tuberculin test. Those showing a positive reaction were sent to one medical ward; those who were tuberculin-negative, to another. Von Pirquet arranged this separation in part so that the infection would not be spread by the children themselves, but chiefly because he wanted to protect those who were free of the disease from becoming infected through contact with adult visitors who might have an active tuberculous focus. We also introduced a ward for juvenile diabetics, which was opened after my return from England with news of the discovery of insulin in 1921. Prior to that time diabetic children had such a short life expectancy that a separate space was not needed. The new ward soon became famous, and children with diabetes were referred from all parts of Europe.

In 1921, I was treating a girl who had a metabolic disorder. Study of the condition showed an abnormality of glycogen storage in the liver and led to the first description of this disease entity. The case was of great interest to research and teaching. The child was treated in one of the medical wards, where she remained for about a year. In order to have the cost of this prolonged hospitalization borne by the institution, approval had to be obtained from the Ministry of Education, which required that status reports be submitted at intervals to show that continuing care was desirable. After the same routine information on this patient had been supplied repeatedly, von Pirquet became weary of the bureaucratic process and said: "We often hear that a dossier has been lost. How would it be if we were to lose this one?" We stopped sending the information.

An interest in psychiatry that began when he was in medical school led to another innovation which proved a milestone in the history of pediatrics. In his opening lecture in Vienna, von Pirquet proposed a psychiatric ward for children. Soon thereafter what he termed a ward for corrective education was added to the *Kinderklinik*. The director of the ward, Professor Erwin Lazar, was a pediatrician who had specialized in psychiatry and served as psychiatric adviser to the city's juvenile court. His staff consisted of an assistant and several nurses who had received specialized training in psychometric techniques. Lazar was a pioneer in this field, and the venture which he and von Pirquet undertook required a good deal of courage. Freud's followers

were found chiefly among a few lay groups; the more conservative medical profession had not accepted his views on psychoanalysis, nor had the general public. Actually, the ostracism of
Freud prior to World War I was based on his psychoanalytical
theories and not, as is sometimes believed, on racial prejudice.
Neither Lazar nor von Pirquet was hostile to Freud's concept.

Von Pirquet had deep interest in the work Lazar was doing
and never failed to listen patiently to the long histories of patients
on his ward during morning rounds. Many of the children were
referred by the police or juvenile court because of behavioral
problems. They were first given medical and psychiatric evaluation, followed by a period of careful observation. Occasionally
the mental abnormality was found to be the result of transitory
somatic disease. Sometimes there were developmental or educational errors which could be corrected by adequate training. In
certain instances, transferral to an institution for mentally retarded children or to a reform school was necessary. Often the
child was normal but had suffered emotional trauma because of
unjust treatment by a parent—an hysterical mother or an alco-
holic father. In each case, treatment was directed toward allevia-
tion of the underlying cause. Von Pirquet was particularly interested in the deviation from normal behavior resulting from
organic brain disease, such as the traits of delinquency that
develop after encephalitis. One of his favorite speculations was
that sudden changes in the blood supply to the brain might cause
oscillations in an individual's psychological state.

What has become a generally accepted practice in pediatrics
was then a daring experiment. Von Pirquet established the first
psychiatric evaluation in a children's hospital in the world and
showed that many sick children could be helped physically
through an understanding of their emotional and environmental
problems. Inevitably the plan was scoffed at and opposed initially,
but as successful results became apparent other pediatric hospitals followed the lead.

Von Pirquet always enjoyed children. When they were present
he was natural and adjusted to their age level. During his rounds
on the roof garden of the *Kinderklinik*, which served as an open-
air ward for children with inactive tuberculosis, he was always
greeted like a friend. Christmas, Carnival, and other holidays
provided welcome opportunity for festivities which he never

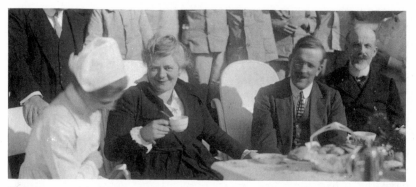

Gathering to mark the introduction of an open-air ward for tuberculosis at the *Kinderklinik*. Left to right: head nurse, Maria, Clemens, and Guido von Pirquet.

missed. Once during a masked ball at Carnival he delighted the children by appearing in the costume of a Chinese mandarin. When he returned from a lecture tour in the United States he taught them the song, "Sing Polly Wolly Doodle All the Day." On the 100th anniversary of Schubert's death, one of the nurses helped the children on the psychiatric ward to prepare a *Schubertfeier* in the composer's honor, to which von Pirquet listened with delight. As Bett commented: "No detail was ever too trivial for his personal attention. He was passionately devoted to children, and it was touching to see him in his klinik surrounded by his little patients, into whose lives he entered with that rare seriousness which is characteristic of the truly great man who has mastered the secret of eternal youth. His scrupulous fairness, courtesy and quiet charm of manner endeared him to all."[8]

Politics held little interest for von Pirquet. He affiliated himself with no political party although he might be considered a forerunner of the liberal reform group which emerged after World War I, or what Bertrand Russell called an "aristocratic liberal." He was, however, moved by the conditions of war to express his views in an open letter. Dated April 10, 1915, the letter was sent to an American friend, Dr. Arthur Howell Gerhard of Philadelphia.

My dear Arthur:

When I was called to Baltimore six years ago to become a professor at Johns Hopkins University, I was often asked: "What will happen in

[8] Walter R. Bett, "Some Paediatric Eponyms. I. Pirquet's Reaction," *Brit. J. Child. Dis.* 26 (1929): 276.

Austria when your old Emperor dies?" I always answered that nothing would change, as all the nationalities of which Austria–Hungary is composed are strongly united not only by dynastic history and tradition, but by geographic necessity. I used to say that I considered the national divergencies only a fashion which would pass with time, just as the religious divergencies of former centuries were smoothed over with time.

The present situation demonstrates the truth of this statement. The fashion of national divergencies has been swept away by the war. Austria–Hungary has been strengthened by the Russian attack just as Germany was strengthened by the French attack in 1870. After this war, our ten different languages will play no more political part than have the twenty principalities of Germany since the Franco-German war. . . .

Russia, since her successful attack on Poland in the eighteenth century, acquired an appetite to extend her autocracy to the southeast of Europe and to devour Turkey in the same way. But Austria–Hungary, which was formed a thousand years ago as a bulwark against eastern invasion, was always the obstacle in the path of Russia. She had to attack Austria–Hungary before she could take possession of the Balkan States. Therefore the Russian proverb originated: "The road to Constantinople leads over Vienna."

In addition, Russia hates Austria because of the bad political example set by the freedom of our nationalities. In the Habsburg monarchy the Hungarians have an absolute self-government, the Poles and the Czechs a practical one, and the smaller nationalities are free to speak, to teach, and to extend their languages and their local patriotism even to a point dangerous to the general welfare of the State. You have traveled enough in Austria–Hungary to remember that the signs in our railway cars are written in four or five different tongues; this is a typical example of the care which the government takes for local and provincial sensibilities.

On the other hand, in Russia the opposite is true. Every effort is expended to assimilate the smaller nationalities. Of her 170 million inhabitants only 44 per cent are Russians; 22 per cent are closely related, but 34 per cent are composed of national groups who speak more than thirty different languages. . . .

Russia hated national independence in Austria–Hungary and at the same time supported the extreme radicals of our Slavic nationalities in order to divide up Austria–Hungary, as European Turkey had been divided, into small national states. For this purpose the aspirations of Servia were very much to Russia's pleasure. The Servians speak the same language as nearly six million inhabitants in the south of our Empire and they made every effort to gain influence in this area. It would be the same as if Mexico were to claim Texas and California from the United States in the name of the Spanish-speaking people living there. The political methods of Servia are those of the most primitive times. You remember how they murdered their former king and you can fancy what an undesirable neighbor they make. An old state like Austria–Hungary, bound by a complicated constitution and on the borders of such a primitive tribe, is in the position of a worthy gentleman being attacked by a rowdy. The gentleman will think of his clothes and of his family; he will hesitate and will try to talk to the rowdy and to pacify him instead of using his fists at once. The gentleman Austria hesitated much more because he knew that the rowdy Servia was a member of a gang, but finally we had to resort to action. . . .

The murder of the governor of Croatia and of Archduke Franz Ferdinand was not the work of crazy individuals, but was plotted by a large organization. This plot had been organized officially in Servia and the bombs and firearms were supplied by Servian officers!

Austria–Hungary knew that Servia was supported by Russia and that this state would use the first opportunity for a fight. But the murder of Archduke Franz Ferdinand seemed too serious an action to be condoned even by Russia. We thought that in such a case the whole world would understand our action and would not interfere. It was a hard decision for our old Emperor. He hated to think of war. Some few years ago, when one of our generals talked of a war against Servia, the Emperor asked: "Have you seen a war yourself?" "No, your Majesty." "Then we had better not talk about it." Franz Joseph in his younger days had been Emperor during the three wars of 1848, 1859, and 1866 and he had decided not to see a fourth one. But after the murder of his nephew he could not help but threaten war, still hoping that Servia would submit. The conditions the Emperor requested from Servia were hard, but not impossible to fulfil. Servia, in fact, was about to give way when the Russian military party interceded. You know the rest: Germany declared to stand by Austria–Hungary; France supported Russia; and England, pretending to aid Belgium, took the opportunity to oppose her trade competitor, Germany.

So the war began. Russia sent the larger part of her army, which had been mobilized months before, against Austria–Hungary, because Austria was her real target. We had a very hard fight against these enormous masses of good-natured Russian peasants, half-wild Cossacks and other irregular eastern tribes. If you should see what crimes these people committed in the territory which they invaded, you would get an impression of medieval, Tataric warfare. All the stories which the English told you about atrocities by the Germans in Belgium seem to have been invented in order to excuse the crimes Russians really did commit. Certainly every war is atrocious. But what the Germans did, when they burned houses in towns where the civil population had fired upon their troops, was absolutely within the hard laws of war. The Germans were severe, but not arbitrary. They knew from the second part of their campaign in France in 1870 that a franc-tireur war could only be suppressed by utmost severity. But the stories about pillaging and murdering, about cutting arms and feet of children, are all rot. This is as contrary to German organization and discipline as if someone would say that I and my assistants were killing the babies in the hospital.

As for the Russians, their behavior varies according to the nature of the troops and the good will and correctness of the individual commanding officers. In some few towns, with an honest general in command, the Russians were orderly; but in most places, especially Bucovina and eastern Galicia, they did all they would and all they could. The worst incidents occurred where the wild southern and Siberian tribes were let loose. . . .

Now a medical point: The Russians not only mobilized millions of soldiers against us, but also billions of small organisms of various kinds. Being a member of the Austrian Board of Health, I know what effort it takes, even in times of peace, to keep down the infections spreading over the border of a state as backward in general sanitation as Russia is. But now we have to deal not with single cases, which we could render inoffensive by isolation, but with scores of infections brought into our territories from Asia. I do not speak of the milliards of fleas and lice, which these people are used to and which our soldiers became accustomed to after some painful weeks. One of my brothers, a retired captain, was on the eastern front in the trenches for six weeks. He told me that practically no one could escape being eaten by vermin.

But there was a more dangerous mobilization of microbes of cholera, smallpox, typhoid fever, and typhus. In the fall, some of our regiments were infected with cholera in Galicia and were practically decimated. Up to now, cholera has not spread inside our lands, but we fear the next summer may bring an increase of this disease. Smallpox is not dangerous for our soldiers, as they are well vaccinated. But our town population is not. We have had already about a thousand cases in Vienna, and the medical faculty is trying very hard to bring about compulsory vaccination. Typhoid fever is usually, as you may remember, an extreme rarity in Vienna. In my hospital, I used to see half a dozen cases in a year; now we are receiving patients daily. The worst of all these diseases is typhus. Up to now, few of our own people have succumbed, but many refugees from Galicia, as well as Russian and Servian prisoners—who are so hard to free from body lice—have been infected. It is a great danger for the visiting physicians. Among many others General Pick, the Surgeon

General of our army in Germany, Professor Jochmann (one of the first authorities on infectious diseases), and recently the Bishop of Linz succumbed to the same infection—each of them after a visit in the prisoners' camp.

Last but not least, an awful invasion of syphilis and gonorrhea has come in with the Russian army in Galicia and Bucovina. You have no idea in what way and in what number women, girls, and even children are ruined. I remember what sentiment it causes in America if one white woman is attacked by a Negro. And here thousands of white women are violated by these Asiatics, under the most terrible circumstances. Many a husband tells that he was forced to watch a dozen Cossacks attacking his wife and his children. . . .

Our soldiers have to fight and they will fight and drive out these eastern invaders. After twenty years the Russian people will be thankful to our soldiers, for the criminal autocracy of Russia will have been eradicated as a result of the terrible war which its policy of expansion has brought forth instead of the education of her illiterate masses and the fertilization of her wonderful soil. The Austrian bulwark will withstand this invasion, as it has withstood the Asiatic invasions for a thousand years.

What could America do? We did not expect any active help from you, but we did expect a sentiment of sympathy in the awful struggle in which we peaceful people have to fight. . . . What we expected of America was sympathy and strict neutrality, and it was with the greatest distress that we saw your merchants send money and ammunition to our enemies. Your Government points out that this is not a breach of neutrality, but only a matter of private enterprise and business. In the same way a usurer will tell you that he breaks no law in lending money to a gambler. This may be a becoming attitude for a small dealer, but not for a nation which could stand above the situation, a nation which could enforce her strong will to do something for the sake of humanity. The sending of ammunition gives no real help to anybody. It will not change the final issue; it only prolongs the war. Each additional shot fired by our enemies means another shot fired by us, means only a prolongation of the manslaughter.

Von Pirquet was wrong in his predictions about the outcome of the war and about the future of nationalism. Grillparzer more accurately described the sequence from humanitarianism through nationalism to bestiality. Von Pirquet did not live long enough to witness the paroxysmal outburst of German nationalism under

Hitler, with atrocities unsurpassed in the history of mankind
That kind of nationalism was alien to the mentality of pre-Hitler
Austria.

The medical complement of the *Kinderklinik* normally consisted of the director and seven assistants. During the period from
1914 to 1918 von Pirquet remained in charge and was permitted to retain one assistant. He chose Bela Schick. The other
six doctors served in the army. Von Gröer, who was also a member
of the staff, was able to remain because he was a Russian citizen
and not subject to military duty. These three men carried on the
work with the help of competent nurses. X-ray and laboratory
studies had to be discontinued; the only research was in the field
of nutrition. Pediatric care was limited to the clinical diagnosis
and treatment of about two hundred patients. Children continued to be admitted, many acutely ill with diphtheria or croup.
Disease increased as refugees flocked into Vienna from the occupied areas, particularly certain parts of Poland, and as the
advance of malnutrition raised the incidence of tuberculosis.
Each of the three pediatricians took his turn at night duty so that
medical coverage was provided at all times. Like other geniuses,
von Pirquet required very little rest. A ten-minute sleep snatched
during the day would send him back to work refreshed.

When war was concluded, all of the former assistants returned
and the work began of reorganizing the *Kinderklinik* and restoring
its role of leadership in pediatrics. I was recommended for the
position of assistant and in the spring of 1919 I had my first conversation with von Pirquet. Although I had attended his lectures
and taken my final examination with him while a medical student,
there had been little personal contact between student and
teacher. The interview—short and precise—was unforgettable.
He wasted no time but came to the point at once. After a brief
explanation he said: "You may start your work immediately, but
a mutual decision will not be reached until the fall." It would be
my duty to reorganize the chemical laboratory, which had been
neglected during the war years. (Up to that time there were no
technicians and normally the laboratory determinations were
carried out by dieners or occasionally by the physicians themselves.)

Reconstruction of the laboratory was aided by funds from the Rockefeller Foundation, which set up an office in the *Kinderklinik*. Professor Jacob Parnas joined the staff for a short time to introduce the newly developed microchemical techniques which provided data vital to an understanding of the diseases of children. In addition to supplying badly needed laboratory equipment and up-to-date X-ray units, the Rockefeller funds supported teaching and built up a library of international literature. Later they endowed fellowships to support scientific study in other parts of Europe or America. Von Pirquet was a trustee of the Rockefeller Foundation and their representative in extending help to Austrian universities. Schick assumed the administrative responsibility.

All of these activities enhanced the international prestige of the Vienna *Kinderklinik* as one of the world centers of pediatrics. Many American physicians received their postgraduate training in Vienna, and the courses were presented in English by the staff of the *Kinderklinik*. The rounds which von Pirquet himself conducted three times a week were so well attended that by the time he arrived at the last bed of the ward, the visitors at the rear of the group were still standing at the first bed. Rounds for students, interns, and residents were conducted every morning by each of the seven assistants in his respective ward; newly admitted patients were seen during afternoon rounds and were visited again in the evening by the assistant on call.

Physicians were not the only guests invited to see the *Kinderklinik* and attend von Pirquet's rounds; other foreigners of distinction were also included. Almost everyone who traveled to Vienna came to visit. I remember, for instance, that Anita Loos came after her novel "Gentlemen Prefer Blondes" had become a best-seller and she received great personal attention. It began to appear as though the Baedeker for Vienna must have listed the *Kinderklinik* with an asterisk. Von Pirquet's rounds had the attraction of a show. It is an old experience that when a crowd forms on the street, more and more people gather around and increase the numbers. The suggestion was occasionally made that we should reduce the number of visitors attending rounds and have the others see the *Klinik* under the guidance of an intern who was multilingual. Nevertheless the system was never changed.

A striking example of the proverbial hospitality of the *Kinder-*

klinik was the welcome extended to a group of English scientists who, under the auspices of the Lister Institute in London and the Medical Research Council of Great Britain, came to Vienna in 1919 for the purpose of studying deficiency diseases.[9] Their isolation during the war years had prevented Vienna scientists from becoming aware of the new work on vitamins. Pirquet was no exception, having been entirely preoccupied with the appalling problems of food deficiency. The British workers were warmly welcomed and were given every assistance in their studies of scurvy in infants and children. Later, they were invited to undertake a joint experimental and clinical investigation of the effect of diet in rickets, a disease which had become almost universal in Viennese infants. A complete ward, with nursing personnel and medical supervision, was placed at their disposal. In addition, they enjoyed the resources of a perfectly equipped X-ray department and the devoted collaboration of the X-ray specialist, Hans Wimberger. At one time or another during the period of the study, which continued until 1922, every department of the *Klinik* and almost every member of the staff assisted in the work. During the three-year period, research was made possible which could hardly have been carried out by guests in any other institution.

Von Pirquet's preface to the monograph reporting this study was a masterpiece of modesty and humility.

When Dr. Chick and her colleagues . . . began their work in my Klinik in 1919, I had little expectation that it would lead to results of much practical value. At that time I was of the opinion that a vitamin deficiency in our ordinary diet was a very exceptional occurrence, as for example in case of infantile scurvy (Möller-Barlow disease). With regard to the aetiology of rickets I held the view that it was an infectious disease, widely prevalent in this part of Europe, producing severe symptoms only in case of those children who possessed special susceptibility as the result of an inherited tendency, of a faulty diet, or of defective general hygiene. I imagined rickets to be a disease comparable to some extent with tuberculosis. . . .

The results of the first two years' work of our British colleagues showed me no reason for changing my opinion . . . but the third year of their work shed new light upon the subject. Convincing results were obtained from a comprehensive series of observations, in which comparison was made of the progress of infants on a diet rich in fat-soluble

[9] Leader of the group was Dame Harriette Chick. Most of the animal experiments were carried out by Miss E. M. M. Hume.

vitamins with those on the diet usual in my Klinik. Of a large series of young infants maintained under exactly similar conditions of excellent general hygiene, rickets developed only in those who received the diet poorer in fat-soluble vitamins, that is without cod-liver oil. Similarly, of children admitted with rickets already developed, healing in winter was observed only in those who received cod-liver oil or light therapy. The facts concerning the production of experimental rickets in animals, the applicability of which to the case of human rickets I had previously doubted, thus proved to be perfectly analogous with those determining the occurrence of the disease in the human infant. Further experimental work showing the development of rickets in rats and puppies upon diets deficient in fat-soluble vitamins destroyed my previous belief in the infectious nature of human rickets, as well as my opinion that infantile scurvy was the only children's disease of practical significance caused by a deficiency of vitamin in the diet.

So much for the theoretical aspect of the matter. From the clinical standpoint there is one thing I should like to mention which my colleagues in their modesty have not made enough of. . . . The two additional wards in which the British workers were largely responsible for the administration and the clinical work were model wards, not only as regards control of the details of feeding, of record keeping, and of tabulation of results, but above all as regards the clinical results obtained. Never in my life have I seen such ideal results in infants' wards. Especially in summer and autumn was one struck by the good colour of the children, who were round and plump and good humoured. Although all were artificially fed, they looked like breast-fed infants enjoying the care of a solicitous mother. . . .

The crucial experiment was thus successfully made. The British workers succeeded with the accuracy of a laboratory experiment, in a city where rickets is extremely prevalent, in maintaining a large number of artificially fed babies free from the disease, and further, in the same wards, were invariably successful in healing children admitted with rickets already developed.

With this the chain of evidence appears to me to be complete that animal experiments upon rickets are applicable also to man, that rickets is a disease of nutrition, and that deficiency of fat-soluble vitamins in diet is an essential cause of the disease.[10]

Only a man of the stature of von Pirquet could have admitted so freely that his previous concept of rickets had been incorrect.

[10] Medical Research Council. Special Report Series No. 77. *Studies of Rickets in Vienna 1919–22.* (Report to the Accessory Food Factors Committee appointed jointly by the Medical Research Council and the Lister Institute.) (London: His Majesty's Stationery Office, 1923.) (Courtesy of H. M. Stationery Office, publisher, London.)

IX

From Anthropometrics to the Pirquet System of Nutrition

The accomplishments of von Pirquet's second period of creativity were in a new field of scientific development, entirely unlike the investigations which had earlier brought him world renown. In his plan of research the emphasis was now shifted away from the diseases responsible for high mortality in children toward what might at first impression appear to be a problem less vital to human survival. Increasing knowledge of the importance of nutrition, however—and the anthropometric studies of this period were a precursor and an essential contribution to his concept of nutrition—has shown that von Pirquet's humanitarian approach had shifted only from individual to race survival.

The first evidence of an interest in nutrition was found in some notes which he wrote in 1909 on the letterhead he used in Baltimore. The study of anthropometry began the next year while he was professor at Breslau. In keeping with his desire to simplify the physical examination of a child and to provide exact data rather than a vague description of findings, he produced an objective standard for determining nutritional status.

Exact measurements of height and weight have little meaning unless they can be related to each other and to the age of a child. To compare the child's age with a table showing average weights for that age gives inadequate and sometimes misleading information. A noted European pediatrician, Camerer, had prepared a table of average heights and weights of German children which became a standard in most pediatric hospitals. For example, if an eleven-year-old boy weighed 38.3 kg. and was 152 cm. in height, Camerer listed his expected weight as 30 kg.; thus the child's actual weight was expressed as +8.3 kg. The boy in question was muscular but rapid growth had made him very lean. With a weight loss of 8.3 kg. he would have been a mere skeleton. The explanation is that his height was 17 cm. greater than Camerer's average of 135 cm. for an eleven-year-old boy; 152 cm. would be the expected height for a boy of approximately fourteen years of age and would correspond with an above-average weight of 41 kg. The boy of eleven was 2.7 kg. below this presumed weight, a deficit compatible with the impression gained from his appearance.

An opposite example was a boy of nine whose height was 120 cm., weight 24.2 kg. On Camerer's scale a nine-year-old boy should weigh 27.5 kg.; thus this child had a deficit of 3.3 kg. His nutritional status was satisfactory but his height corresponded to that of an eight-year-old boy who should weigh 25 kg. Therefore his weight was approximately that to be expected for his height. From such considerations von Pirquet concluded that a child's weight should be compared with his height rather than with the average weight for his age. For the majority of children whose build is approximately normal, height can be a satisfactory guide to nutritional status, but errors occur when growth is retarded or when the head is particularly large.

The question then arose of whether a child's desired weight should be determined on the basis of the height for a different age group. Children of the same age have approximately the same proportions; as they become older the proportions agree more closely with height than with age. If a newborn boy 50 cm. in length and weighing 3.4 kg. were to be placed in a cube, each side of which equaled the length of the child, thirty-six newborn infants of that size could be accommodated in the cube provided their specific gravity was equal to that of water. A twelve-year-old boy, 140 cm. in height and 35 kg. in weight, occupies a much smaller volume in relation to his length. A similar cube to accommodate his height would contain 2,744,000 cc., of which the child would occupy only 35,000 cc.; seventy-eight twelve-year-old boys would find room in such a cube.

A boy's height increases more than is to be expected from his gain in weight, particularly in the first three years. In that period the ratio of cubed length to weight increases from 36.76 to 54.71, an increment of 6 per year. Thereafter, until the end of the sixteenth year, the stretching increases at a less rapid rate from 54.71 to 88.22, an average of less than 3 per year.

For girls the ratio in the first three years is exactly the same as for boys; thereafter growth is more intensive up to the twelfth year, when the ratios again correspond. The onset of sexual maturity, together with gain in weight, is manifest two years earlier in girls. In both sexes the constancy of the ratio is striking during the sixth year, when weight and height increase uniformly. A child's body structure is geometrically similar at five and six years of age.

Using Camerer's figures, von Pirquet compiled a simple table, based on height rather than on body proportions, which gave the age and weight of an average boy and girl for each centimeter of body length (Table I). An example will illustrate how height and weight can be evaluated by means of the table. A boy of fourteen years and six months has a height of 155 cm. and a weight of 40.5 kg. His height corresponds to that of a boy of fourteen years and eight months whose weight would be 43.6 kg. His actual weight is 3.1 kg. below that estimated for his height. At fourteen years and six months the boy's height is expected to be 154 cm. His measurements are recorded as −3.1 kg. and +1 cm. Considerable changes occur in the ratio of height to weight during childhood, the ratio for the newborn being more than twice that for a fourteen-year-old child.[1]

A few years later, from the relationship between heart, pulse rate, and body weight, von Pirquet discovered accidentally that the sitting height was closely related to the cube root of body weight. While studying the growth of the body and of its organs in 1914, he made graphic analyses based on clinical and animal data which several investigators had compiled for the heart weight, pulse frequency, and linear growth of the body. He became interested in the relationship between the weight of the heart and the pulse rate. To obtain a linear measurement of the side of the heart he took the cube root of heart weight, assuming its specific gravity to be the same as that of water. The duration of pulse, or interval from the peak of one heart beat to the peak of the next, is a reciprocal value of the pulse rate per minute. If an adult's pulse rate is 60 per minute, the duration of the pulse is 1 second. Von Pirquet estimated that the duration of a man's pulse could be expressed by a figure approximately 4/30 that of the side of his heart. If a heart were to weigh 216 gm. its cube root would be 6; thus the side of the heart would be 6 cm. long. The duration of each pulse beat would be 4/30 of 6 or 0.8 second.

[1] "Eine einfache Tafel zur Bestimmung von Wachstum und Ernährungszustand bei Kindern." *Ztschr. f. Kinderheilk.* 6 (1913): 253.

Table 1. Age, Length, and Weight of Children*

Boys			Girls	
Weight (kg.)	Age	Length (cm.)	Age	Weight (kg.)
3.48	At birth	49	At birth	3.24
3.7		50		3.5
3.9		51		3.7
4.1		52		3.9
4.4	1 mo.	53	1 mo.	4.1
4.7		54		4.3
5.0		55		4.5
5.3	2 mo.	56	2 mo.	4.8
5.6		57		5.1
5.9		58		5.4
6.2	3 mo.	59		5.7
6.5		60	3 mo.	6.0
6.8		61		6.3
7.0	4 mo.	62		6.6
7.3		63	4 mo.	6.9
7.6	5 mo.	64		7.1
7.9		65	5 mo.	7.4
8.2	6 mo.	66		7.6
8.5	7 mo.	67	6 mo.	7.8
8.7		68		8.0
8.9	8 mo.	69	7 mo.	8.2
9.2	9 mo.	70	8 mo.	8.5
9.5	10 mo.	71	9 mo.	8.8
9.7		72	10 mo.	9.1
9.9	11 mo.	73	11 mo.	9.4
10.20	1 yr.	74	1 yr.	9.7
10.45	1 mo.	75	1 mo.	9.95
		76	2 mo.	10.20

Boys			Girls	
Weight (kg.)	Age	Length (cm.)	Age	Weight (kg.)
10.70	2 mo.	77	4 mo.	10.45
10.95	4 mo.	78	5 mo.	10.70
11.20	5 mo.	79	6 mo.	10.95
11.45	6 mo.	80	7 mo.	11.20
11.70	7 mo.	81	8 mo.	11.45
11.95	8 mo.	82	10 mo.	11.70
12.20	10 mo.	83	11 mo.	11.95
12.45	11 mo.	84	2 yr.	12.20
12.70	2 yr.	85	2 mo.	12.45
12.95	2 mo.	86	3 mo.	12.70
13.20	3 mo.	87	5 mo.	12.95
13.45	5 mo.	88	6 mo.	13.20
13.70	6 mo.	89	8 mo.	13.45
13.95	8 mo.	90	9 mo.	13.70
14.20	9 mo.	91	11 mo.	13.95
14.45	11 mo.	92	3 yr.	14.20
14.70	3 yr.	93	2 mo.	14.45
15.00	2 mo.	94	4 mo.	14.70
15.3	4 mo.	95	6 mo.	14.95
15.6	6 mo.	96	8 mo.	15.30
15.9	8 mo.	97	10 mo.	15.45
16.2	10 mo.	98	4 yr.	15.70
16.5	4 yr.	99	2 mo.	15.95
16.8	2 mo.	100	5 mo.	16.20
17.1	5 mo.	101	7 mo.	16.45
17.4	7 mo.	102	10 mo.	16.70
17.7	10 mo.	103	5 yr.	17.0
18.0	5 yr.	104	3 mo.	17.5

Table I—Continued

Boys		Length (cm.)	Girls	
Weight (kg.)	Age		Age	Weight (kg.)
18.5	2 mo.	105	6 mo.	18.0
19.0	5 mo.	106	9 mo.	18.5
19.5	7 mo.	107	6 yr.	19.0
20.0	10 mo.	108	2 mo.	19.3
20.5	6 yr.	109	4 mo.	19.7
21.0	2 mo.	110	6 mo.	20.0
21.4	4 mo.	111	8 mo.	20.3
21.8	6 mo.	112	10 mo.	20.7
22.2	8 mo.	113	7 yr.	21.0
22.6	10 mo.	114	2 mo.	21.4
23.0	7 yr.	115	5 mo.	21.8
23.4	2 mo.	116	7 mo.	22.2
23.8	5 mo.	117	10 mo.	22.6
24.2	7 mo.	118	8 yr.	23.0
24.6	10 mo.	119	2 mo.	23.4
25.0	8 yr.	120	5 mo.	23.8
25.5	2 mo.	121	7 mo.	24.2
26.0	5 mo.	122	10 mo.	24.6
26.5	7 mo.	123	9 yr.	25.0
27.0	10 mo.	124	2 mo.	25.4
27.5	9 yr.	125	5 mo.	25.8
28.0	2 mo.	126	7 mo.	26.2
28.5	5 mo.	127	10 mo.	26.6
29.0	7 mo.	128	10 yr.	27.0
29.5	10 mo.	129	2 mo.	27.4
30.0	10 yr.	130	5 mo.	27.8
30.5	2 mo.	131	7 mo.	28.2
31.0	5 mo.	132	10 mo.	28.6
31.5	7 mo.	133	11 yr.	29.0
32.0	10 mo.	134	2 mo.	29.5
32.5	11 yr.	135	4 mo.	30.0
33.0	2 mo.	136	6 mo.	30.5
33.5	5 mo.	137	8 mo.	31.0
34.0	7 mo.	138	10 mo.	31.5
34.5	10 mo.	139	12 yr.	32.0
35.0	12 yr.	140	2 mo.	32.7
35.5	2 mo.	141	3 mo.	33.4
36.0	5 mo.	142	5 mo.	34.1
36.5	7 mo.	143	7 mo.	34.8
37.0	10 mo.	144	9 mo.	35.5
37.5	13 yr.	145	10 mo.	36.2
38.0	2 mo.	146	13 yr.	37.0
38.6	4 mo.	147	2 mo.	37.8
39.2	6 mo.	148	3 mo.	38.6
39.8	8 mo.	149	5 mo.	39.4
40.4	10 mo.	150	7 mo.	40.3
41.0	14 yr.	151	9 mo.	41.2
41.6	2 mo.	152	10 mo.	42.1
42.3	4 mo.	153	14 yr.	43.0
43.0	6 mo.	154	2 mo.	44.0
43.6	8 mo.	155	5 mo.	45.0
44.3	10 mo.	156	7 mo.	46.0
45.0	15 yr.	157	10 mo.	47.0
45.7	2 mo.	158	15 yr.	48.0
46.4	3 mo.	159	6 mo.	50.0
47.1	5 mo.	160	16 yr.	52.0

*Compiled by von Pirquet from the average figures of von Camerer. *From:* "Eine einfache Tafel zur Bestimmung von Wachstum und Ernahrungszustand bei Kindern," *Ztschr. f. Kinderheilk.* 6 (1913): 260. (Courtesy of Springer-Verlag, Heidelberg.)

By reversing the process he calculated heart weight from duration of pulse. If the pulse beat is 70 per minute its duration is 60/70 second.

$$\text{Heart weight} = \left(\frac{30}{4} \times \frac{60}{70}\right)^3 = \left(\frac{1,800}{280}\right)^3 = 6.43^3 = 267 \text{ gm.}$$

With a pulse rate of 60 per minute the heart weight would be 422 gm.; for an eight-year-old child with a pulse rate of 90, the heart would weigh 125 gm.

Other investigators had stated that the heart weight of an adult male ranged from 297 to 386 gm., that of an adult female from 221 to 294 gm., and that of a nine-year-old boy about 108 gm. Von Pirquet's results agreed approximately with the established values. He recognized, however, that this was an impractical method of determining heart weight because the pulse could be counted accurately only with the subject at complete rest, under the conditions required for basal metabolism, and such a condition was almost impossible to attain in a child. Much simpler was to estimate heart weight as 0.5 per cent of total body weight. The significance of the findings lay in the fact that the duration of pulse bore direct relation to the cube root of the heart weight and thus to the cube root of body weight.

Two years later he became aware that the number of centimeters of sitting height and the number of seconds required for 100 pulse beats were almost identical for children whose sitting heights ranged between 60 and 80 cm. (Table 2). In infants a deviation occurred, most pronounced in the newborn, but during childhood the pulse rate per minute could be estimated from sitting height more accurately than it could be counted. Von Pirquet explained the theoretical significance of this relationship by saying that the duration of pulse is a function of the first power, whereas the heart rate, and hence its volume, is proportionate to body weight, a third power.

In a given period of time the volume of blood pumped through the heart is the same as the stroke volume of the heart multiplied by the pulse rate. The turnover of energy in a healthy individual during a similar period of time is proportional to the blood volume with its accumulated oxygen, carbon dioxide, and nutrients, and hence is proportional to the heart volume multiplied by pulse

Table 2. Theoretical Relation of Sitting Height, Heart Weight,
and Duration of Pulse

	Boys		Girls	
Sitting height (cm.)	Side of heart (cube root of heart weight) (cm.)	Duration of 100 pulse beats (sec.)	Side of heart (cube root of heart weight) (cm.)	Duration of 100 pulse beats (sec.)
80	6.0	80	5.68	75.6
75	5.65	75.3	5.33	71
70	5.25	70	5.03	67
65	4.85	64.6	4.75	63
60	4.6	61.2	4.5	60
55	4.35	58	4.3	57
50	4.08	54.3	4.0	53
45	3.68	49	3.6	48
40	3.33	44.4	3.28	43.6
35	2.97	39.3	2.97	39.5

From: "Pulsfrequenz und Sitzhöhe." *Ztschr. f. Kinderheilk.* 38 (1924): 302. (Courtesy of Springer-Verlag, Heidelberg.)

rate. Consequently, because pulse rate is a reciprocal of duration of pulse

$$\text{Turnover of energy} \simeq \frac{\text{Volume of heart}}{\text{Duration of pulse}}.$$

Since the heart volume is in proportion to its weight, and duration of pulse to the cube root of the heart weight, turnover of energy must be a function of the second power.

$$\text{Turnover of energy} \simeq \frac{\text{Heart weight}}{\sqrt[3]{\text{Heart weight}}} = \text{Heart weight}^{2/3}.$$

It was at this point that von Pirquet formed his conception of the significance of the sitting height, when he pointed out that the body weight (in grams) of a muscular adult was approximately equal to one-tenth of the cube of the sitting height.[2] As the heart weight is proportional to the body weight and the duration of pulse to the sitting height, therefore:

$$\text{Turnover of energy} \simeq \frac{\text{Volume of heart}}{\text{Duration of pulse}} \propto \frac{\text{Sitting height}^3}{\text{Sitting height}}.$$

[2] "Sitzhöhe und Körpergewicht," *Ztschr. f. Kinderheilk.* 14 (1916): 211.

Thus the turnover of energy is proportional to the square of the sitting height.

To demonstrate how his theories could be applied, he prepared a series of tables which compared sitting height and pulse rate for the newborn, older infants and children, and adults.[3] Even when calculations were based on sitting height rather than total height, he was able to substantiate his early findings.

From comparison of pulse rate and sitting height, von Pirquet's thoughts followed a tangent which led first to the relation of metabolism to sitting height and then to the significance of the square of the sitting height in human nutrition. After applying this concept to nutrition of the individual and of masses of individuals, he eventually returned to the circle from which the tangent had diverged.

The sitting height, or height of the trunk, is ascertained by measuring the distance between the horizontal seat on which the body rests and a horizontal board on top of the head. This measure is not quite exact, for it depends upon the position of the spine and the degree of compression of the intervertebral disks, and hence it varies with the position of the body as well as with the period of the day. The same objections, however, apply to standing height. No measurement which includes a joint can be mathematically exact, but if the child sits as erect as possible the limits of error will fall within 1 cm. Young infants are measured in the horizontal position, from a vertical board pressed against the seat to another placed against the head. A few examples of von Pirquet's anthropometric material were published several years later:

	Standing height (cm.)	Sitting height (cm.)	Weight (kg.)
Fetus (about 70 days old)	26.6	17	0.35
Newborn	50.5	32	2.9
Eight-year-old child	116.0	66	22.3
Adult	177.0	93	73.3

[3] "Pulsfrequenz und Sitzhöhe," *Ztschr. f. Kinderheilk.* 38 (1924): 301. This work was not published in its entirety until after it had been presented at the International Physiological Congress in Edinburgh in 1923.

From fetus to adult the standing height advances from 26.6 to 177 cm., or at a ratio of 1:6.6. The sitting height shows a somewhat smaller variation, 1:5.5. The weight, on the other hand, ranges from 350 to 73,300 gm., a ratio of 1:209. The largest factor in the difference between standing height and sitting height is the relatively short legs of the fetus and the newborn infant.

Another table shows the ratio of the cube root of weight to sitting height:

	Fetus	Newborn	Eight-year-old	Adult
Weight (gm.)	350	2,900	22,300	73,300
Cube root of above	7.04	14.3	28.1	41.9
Sitting height	17.0	32.0	66.0	93.0
Ratio of $\sqrt[3]{\text{weight}}$: sitting height	0.415	0.446	0.426	0.450

This ratio varies only from 0.415 for fetus to 0.450 for adult, or at the rate of 100:108, whereas the sitting-height ratio is 100:547 and the weight ratio is 100:20,900. Von Pirquet found that he could show the relationship without computing the ratio if, instead of the cube root of actual weight, he took that of the weight multiplied by 10. This cube root differed but little from the sitting height: 15.2 and 17, 90.1 and 93, as shown in the following table:

	Fetus	Newborn	Eight-year-old	Adult
Weight (gm.) × 10	3,500	29,000	223,000	733,000
Cube root of above	15.2	30.7	60.5	90.1
Sitting height	17.0	32.0	66.0	93.0
Ratio	89.0	96.0	92.0	97.0

The variation in ratio from 89 to 97 is further equalized by the fact that the thin fetus and the thin eight-year-old boy show similar values, as do also the robust newborn and the adult of average stature. Hence a close relationship exists between sitting height and weight.

A cube of which one side is the sitting height—in which the human being could sit upright—if filled with water would represent ten times the weight of the human body. In other words, this cube could hold ten closely packed persons. Von Pirquet expressed this law by saying that the cube root of ten times the weight in grams approximately equals the sitting height in centimeters.

$$\sqrt[3]{10 \text{ times weight}} = \text{Sitting height}$$

or

$$\frac{\sqrt[3]{10 \text{ times weight}}}{\text{Sitting height}} = \frac{100}{100}.$$

If the weight is greater than average, the ratio will be more than 100/100. For instance, if a man of 90 cm. sitting height weighed 72.9 kg., his weight would exactly correspond to the rule, as the cube root of 729,000 is 90. But if he weighed 82.9 kg. the formula would be

$$\frac{\sqrt[3]{829,000}}{90} = \frac{104}{100}.$$

If he weighed only 62.9 kg., the formula would be

$$\frac{\sqrt[3]{629,000}}{90} = \frac{95}{100}.$$

This formula for comparing sitting height and weight was made easier to remember by an acronym which he devised to designate his index of nutritional status:

P stands for Pondus, the body weight in grams. *Pe* recalls the fact that we have to take not the simple weight, but pondus *decies*, ten times the weight. *Li* tells us that the weight must be converted into a linear function by taking the cube root of it. *Di* means division and *Si*, sitting height. The word, therefore, is *pelidisi*. We say the pelidisi of this man of 90 cm. sitting height and 72.9 kilograms is 100; if he puts on 10 kilograms more weight, it will be 104; if he loses 10 kilograms, it will be 95.

It would be asking too much of the physician to estimate the cube root of the weight of every patient and afterward perform a division. But this calculation is very easy if he uses a table, where he has only to look for the headings and go down a line of figures until he finds the weight. At the angle he then finds the pelidisi. . . .

Notwithstanding the growth of the extremities and their corresponding increase in weight, the relation between sitting height and total height of the body remains uniform for fetus or adult. The pelidisi index may range from less than 90 for a thin child to approximately 100 for one with a good deal of fatty tissue. For adults an extra 5 points must be allowed for musculature, so that the range might be from less than 95 to more than 105. Because the variations in ratio are so similar, the pelidisi can be used to express the nutritional status of any individual.[4]

This subject no longer seems complicated, now that both pediatricians and parents are familiar with nutritional charts, but it became clear largely through the efforts of von Pirquet. He was the pioneer in devising a simple method of expressing a child's nutritional status. Later formulas and approaches followed the lines which he laid down. The Camerer–Pirquet figures were— and are today—used at the Vienna *Kinderklinik*. There von Pirquet's methods were taught to pediatricians from all over the world, including Harold C. Stuart and the Bakwins, whose percentile charts and tables are now popular in the United States. Their figures, however, are based on the proportions of American children, which differ from those of German children.

With a criterion at hand for measuring a child's nutritional status, von Pirquet was ready to begin his work of simplifying and standardizing the values for infant nutrition. This was not, to be sure, his first consideration of the subject. In the notes which he had written while in Baltimore, mentioned previously, he had defined what he called a nutritional unit as that amount of food containing one large unit of heat (one large calorie), and had expressed the formulas then in use in terms of his nutritional units. For example, human milk and cow's milk, each having a caloric value of 700 small calories per gram, in his system were given the value of 1.43 nutritional units.

His tendency to express observations, reactions, and dynamic processes through formulas or charts was evident even earlier. In 1908 he had stated: "This presentation [i.e., the graphic analysis of a phenomenon] was for me not accidental, but rather the result of preliminary studies over many years. . . . " A little later, as a hobby, he began to form acronyms by replacing numbers with selected combinations of vowels and consonants. Because spoken numbers are easily misunderstood, he recommended that letter combinations, or what he called *Zahlenlaute* (sounds for

[4] *An Outline of the Pirquet System of Nutrition* (Philadelphia: W. B. Saunders Co., 1922). (Courtesy of W. B. Saunders Co., publisher, Philadelphia.)

numerals), be applied wherever a number was not part of a calculation but had spoken significance only, as in telephoning; in railway and telegraph service; for doctors describing the size, shape, color, and other properties of skin reactions; in international business; and even for giving commands in the army. The latter had particular application for the Austro-Hungarian army with its thirteen different nationalities. Today such acronyms as radar, NATO, and UNESCO are in constant use. Sometimes, of course, more time is spent in deciphering the acronym than would be needed to write out the entire words.

Moreover, in 1911 he had been asked to complete an unfinished abstract of Theodor Escherich's lectures on infant nutrition. Here von Pirquet stressed the importance of adequate nutrition in health and disease. He calculated the nutritional requirement empirically from the volume of breast milk taken by a healthy infant. The work was based in part upon student lectures which he himself had given. Before his time a little information about calories had been included in the physiology course, but medical students gained no scientific idea of nutrition. The main principles involved were now compressed into eight charts (Figs. 16 and 17 are samples). Emphasizing the interdependence of weight curve and intake of food, these charts form the skeleton of von Pirquet's nutritional concepts. Although not directly related to the Nem System, this study used a similar quantitative approach.

Evidence of all of the activities mentioned in this chapter appears in the system of nutrition,[5] where von Pirquet's interest in body measurements and their relation to nutritional requirements was combined with a new standard to replace the calorie. Work on this subject became intensified after the eruption of World War I, when scarcity of food and increasing morbidity and mortality from tuberculosis foretold widespread starvation in Central Europe. In 1917 the first volume of the Pirquet system of nutrition was published, followed by the second and third volumes in 1919 and the fourth in 1920.[6] Complicated data and charts depict the scientific material upon which the system rests, and the German volumes are too detailed for most medical

---

[5] Von Pirquet did not identify his ideas as a theory or a concept, but as a *system* of nutrition. In this he was like Linné, a great organizer in another science, who established a new—and artificial—system of botany which is still valid.

[6] *System der Ernährung* (Berlin: Julius Springer, 1917–20).

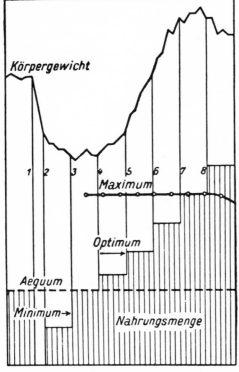

Fig. 16. Minimum, aequum, optimum, and maximum levels of food intake. (*Korpergewicht*, body weight. *Nahrungsmenge*, quantity of food.) *From:* Nobel, E., Pirquet, C., and Wagner, R. *The Nutrition of Healthy and Sick Infants and Children*, transl. B. M. Gasul (2d ed.; Philadelphia: F. A. Davis Co., 1929), p. 64. (Courtesy of F. A. Davis, Philadelphia.)

practitioners. Numerous explanatory articles and graphic material were later published by von Pirquet and his coworkers, including a textbook on nutrition of the masses written in collaboration with Mayerhofer[7] and another by Nobel, Pirquet, and Wagner on nutrition of children.[8]

One of the clearest descriptions of the system was written in English. As Silliman lecturer on modern pediatrics at Yale

[7] *Lehrbuch der Volksernährung nach dem Pirquet'schen System* (Vienna: Urban and Schwarzenberg, 1920). (With E. Mayerhofer.)

[8] *The Nutrition of Healthy and Sick Infants and Children*, transl. B. M. Gasul (2d ed.; Philadelphia: F. A. Davis Co., 1929). (With E. Nobel and R. Wagner.)

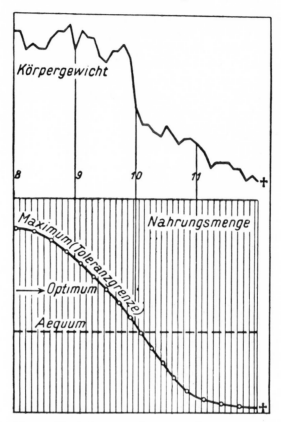

Fig. 17. Death due to continuous overfeeding. (*Toler-anzgrenze*, tolerance limit.) *From:* Nobel, E., Pirquet, C., and Wagner, R. *The Nutrition of Healthy and Sick Infants and Children*, transl. B. M. Gasul (2d ed.; Philadelphia: F. A. Davis Co., 1929), p. 67. (Courtesy of F. A. Davis, Philadelphia.)

University in the winter of 1921–22, von Pirquet devoted several of his lectures to the subject of nutrition. Complying with the requests of many friends, he prepared a small book based on the lecture material. To this he added a bibliographic list of publications on nutrition for the years 1917 to 1922, the *nem* (*n*utritional *e*quivalent of *m*ilk) values of principal foods, a table of pelidisi, and a description of the relationship between body measurements and nutrition.[9]

In the Europe of fifty years ago the German physiologist Max Rubner was highly respected and pediatricians looked to him for

[9] Von Pirquet, *The Pirquet System of Nutrition.*

fundamental concepts of nutrition. Rubner believed that energy requirements should be determined from body surface rather than body weight, and that the nutritional state depended upon the amount of heat given off by an animal at rest and fasting. His theory was that body heat is generated by oxidation of the reserve substances of the body, particularly fat, and depends upon two factors. First, it is a by-product of the oxidation necessary to maintain life functions, such as action of the heart and lungs or secretion of the glands. Second, in a cold environment it is augmented by the more or less spontaneous movements which are an individual's attempt to maintain a uniform internal temperature and avoid extreme cooling of the body.

Von Pirquet agreed with Rubner that nutritional requirements should be based on body surface, but differed in the method of calculation. He reasoned that, although valuable physiological conclusions could be drawn by testing individuals deprived of food and at rest, normally man's desire for food and sleep is satisfied. Rubner's experimental requirements could most nearly be approximated in the individual working with his brain, but an entirely different type of oxidation occurs in the active, growing child or the manual laborer. Von Pirquet continued: "As a rule the human organism takes in far larger masses of food than suffice for heating its furnace and maintaining the body temperature. The workingman does not eat for the purpose of keeping his body temperature from falling. On the contrary, he possesses a superabundance of heat which he seeks to eliminate by evaporation." Therefore von Pirquet based his own theory of nutrition not on the amount of heat given off by the body, but on *the amount of oxidizable intake in the form of food:*

The law that the production of heat corresponds to a surface and not to a cube has, long before Rubner, been expressed by Rameaux in 1838, and by Bergman in 1847; the theory that the output of heat is not the real standard has been brought forward by H. von Hoesslin in 1888. The absorbed oxygen, this author pointed out, is proportionate to the amount of oxygen which is circulating in the body. That amount has a relation to the cross-section surface of the blood-vessels, and this again is proportionate to the two-thirds power of the weight. Also, the amount of food taken in by the body is related to a theoretical intestinal surface, which surface again is related to the surface of a cross-section of the body, and, therefore, to a two-thirds power of weight. Without knowing of the work of Hoesslin, I myself had come to similar conclusions as to the importance of the two-thirds power of the weight, and I tried to find a way of easy calculation for a surface which we could take as representing the absorbing surface through which the food taken in the body had to pass. As I knew that the sitting height stood in a constant and simple relation to the cube root of the weight, the two-thirds power of the weight could be easily calculated by taking the square of the sitting height. As this surface interested me in regard to the intake, I had to find out whether or not we could bring it into direct relation with the absorbing surface of the intestines, and this could be done in a very simple way.

Henning had found in 1881 that in children as well as in adults the length of the intestinal canal directly corresponds to the sitting height, a thing which seems to us now a matter of course, as every part of the trunk in a well-proportioned individual will be proportionate to the length of the trunk. But he also had found a very simple relation; the length of the intestinal canal on an average equals ten times the sitting height. Direct measurements of the surface of the intestines gave for the undilated canal of an adult about 5000 sq. cm.; for the dilated, about 10,000 sq. cm.; if we take a medium of 7500 sq. cm., this corresponds to an average circumference of about one-tenth of the sitting height. We can, therefore, have a conception of the absorbing surface in multiplying ten times the sitting height by one-tenth of the sitting height, or, in other words, we take the square of the sitting height as a symbol of the absorbing surface. . . .

By comparing the intake of mammals of distinctly different sizes, von Pirquet showed that the two-thirds power of the weight had a true relation to the intake of food:

	Weight (gm.)	Intake per day (nem)	Nem per 1000 gm.	Intestinal surface (10 times weight)$^{2/3}$	Daily intake (nem per sq. cm. of intestinal surface)
Rat	181	58	320	148	0.392
Newborn child	2,200	336	152	784	0.429
Adult	61,400	3,063	50	7,230	0.423
Ox	632,100	15,200	24	34,200	0.445
Highest figure divided by lowest figure	3,500	261	13.3	231	1.14

The ox has a weight 3500 times the weight of the rat, but the food he takes in is not 3500 times more, but only 261 times;[10] compared to weight, the rat eats 13.3 times more than the ox. It is apparent that the intake corresponds much closer to the two-thirds power of [10 times] the weight, as here the relation of ox to rat is only 231 to 1. But we see the clearest expression of the law in the last column, which expresses the relation of the daily intake to the intestinal surface: The rat takes 0.392 food units per square centimeter, the baby, 0.429, the adult, 0.423, the ox, 0.445; the division of the highest by the lowest figure gives only 1.14 compared to 231 for surface, 261 for intake, and 3500 for weight.

Having found these simple ways of comparison, I spent about two years in examining the spontaneous intake of children and adults, and comparing these figures with the two-thirds power of the weight and the square of the sitting height. More than 10,000 single day experiments have been used for the calculation. . . . The correspondence was remarkably close, and the method of using the square of the sitting height proved to be more satisfactory for practical use because it has the advantage over the two-thirds power of the weight in that it does not depend on the accessory surplus or lack of fat tissue and muscles, but is rather related to an ideal status of nutrition that corresponds to the skeleton.

Von Pirquet next spent about two years devising simple principles, based upon the square of the sitting height, which could be applied to the nutritional needs of individuals.

In the Silliman lectures he also discussed his reasons for replacing the calorie by his own nutritional unit, the nem. He defined the nem as the nutritive, combustible value of 1 gm. of average human milk having a theoretical content of 1.7 per cent protein, 3.7 per cent fat, and 6.7 per cent milk sugar. The nem could also be applied to standard cow's milk having 3.3 per cent protein, 3.7 per cent fat, and 5 per cent milk sugar. He reasoned that although milk varied greatly, especially in its fat content, nevertheless it was as appropriate to take a theoretical average as a standard for milk as to consider horsepower a standard for machines even though each horse has different strength.

[10] Biologists explain this finding when they state that the volume of a body grows as the cube of its linear dimensions; the surface grows as the square. The rat, which has a large surface in proportion to its mass, expends a great deal of energy in replacing the heat lost from the surface and hence must eat larger quantities of food in proportion to weight than the ox.

The standard milk I chose has a simple relation to the caloric system, having 667 small available calories in 1 gram, or 667 large calories in 1 kilogram; 2000 small calories, therefore 2 large calories, equal 3 nem, or one large calory equals 1.5 nem.

But why not take the calories as they are? Why introduce a new standard? There are several reasons for this. The calorie, which dates from Lavoisier's time, has been very well defined for the physicist as the amount of heat necessary to raise the temperature of 1 gram of water 1°C.—this is the so-called small calory. The large calory raises the temperature of 1000 grams 1°C. This is clear when a bomb calorimeter is used, but not if the combustion takes place in a living being. A portion of the food ingested is not available for heat production, since a fraction of it passes off from the body undigested. Some of the physiologists distinguish, therefore, the net from the raw calory, some discount the unburned part in the feces, some discount also the unburned output in the urine—the fact is, that every one of the greater schools of physiology has its own definition, and, therefore, arrives at a different caloric value for the food-stuffs of ordinary use.

What we need is a simple physiologic unit. The calory does not supply it. Coal, for instance, is wonderfully rich in calories if you burn it in an oven, but it has no food value, because it passes the intestinal canal without being absorbed. If you burn leafy sprigs in a calorimeter the caloric value may be large, but if you feed the same to cattle you discover not only that the animals are unable to avail themselves of the heat value but also that they actually lose weight because of the work of mastication and of transformation of the sprigs into a pulpy mass that can pass through the intestines. Because of this the agriculturists have long ago abandoned the caloric system. They use different physiologic units of comparison, of which, to my mind, the starch unit of Kellner is the best. It compares the amount of fat produced by 1 kilogram of various food-stuffs given as a surplus to a minimum ration with the amount of fat produced by ingestion of 1 kilogram of water-free starch as a standard. Both unit and point of comparison seemed not to be applicable to human beings, for we do not use water-free starch, and our object is not to produce lard. I thought milk much more appropriate for a practical unit, as it is the first food we give to human beings. During childhood we substitute slowly other materials for it. Moreover, it contains all the important food-stuffs, the combustibles (fat and carbohydrates), the structural elements (water and salt), and the proteins which can be used both as structural elements and as combustibles, and finally, the vitamins.

This milk unit is used as a metric unit, and is combined with the Latin prefixes for metric fractions, and with the Greek prefixes for multiples of the unit:

A decinem means one-tenth of a nem, or the nutritive value of 1 decigram of milk, 0.1 gm., and is written 1 dn.

A centinem is written 1 cn., and represents 0.01 gm.

A millinem is written 1 mn., and represents 0.001 gm.

These smaller units are used only in the calculation of the food intake per square centimeter in its relation to the nutritional surface. For instance, in the above example [p. 136], we would say the baby's intake was 4.29 decinem per square centimeter, or 42.9 centinem, or 429 millinem.

In the practical use of food-stuffs we have to make use of the larger units, namely, the multiples with Greek prefixes:

A dekanem (Dn.) means 10 nem.

A hektonem (Hn.) means 100 nem. This unit is used in the composition of a recipe for a certain dish, or of the day's program for one person or family.

A kilonem (Kn.) means 1000 nem. We use it in buying food-stuffs for a family, or making recipes for a large number.

A tonnenem (Tn.), finally, represents the food value of 1 metric ton of milk: 1000 Kn., or 1,000,000 nem. We use it in wholesale nutrition. . . .

The tonnenem was applied in mass feeding studies by the American Relief Administration European Children's Fund. In Austria 400,000 meals were served daily, each of 1 Kn., or a daily total of 400 Tn. To supply this amount of food for twelve days would require a train of 60 cars, each carrying 16 metric tons, or a total of 960 metric tons.

The food values of all articles used for human food should be determined by substituting a given quantity of the article for milk. This method is being worked out for some food-stuffs used in early infancy, but it will take years to finish this experiment for the very many food-stuffs we use for adults. Meantime we use a chemical analysis of the food, discount the percentage of combustibles lost in the urine and in the stools, and translate grams and calories into nem.

To shorten the chemical analysis I devised simple methods of examination, based on the testing of dry substances, fat, and ashes, which are easy to apply, and give results that are satisfactory for practical use. Cow's milk, for instance, has to be examined as to its fat content alone, and bread as to its content in dry substance. . . .

I give some of the most important food-stuffs in the following table, which gives at the same time the weight of 1 hektonem in grams: If 1 gram of flour has a food value of 5 nem, 20 grams will contain 100 nem, or 1 hektonem. The "hektonem-weight" of flour, therefore, is 20.

Nem in 1 gm.		Hektonem weight
13⅓	Pure fat, oil	7.5
12	Butter	8.5
10	Bacon	10
6	Sugar, cocoa	16.7
5	Wheat flour, oat flour, biscuit, rice, ham, fresh fat meat, cheese, syrup, honey	20
4	White bread	25
3⅓	Dark bread	30
2.5	Fresh meat, eggs	40
1.25	Potatoes	80
1	Milk, green peas	100
0.67	Fresh fruit	150
0.5	Skimmed milk	200
0.4	Turnips, spinach, cabbage, cauliflower, fresh mushrooms	250
0.2	Lettuce, cucumbers	500

A good breakfast for an adult, with a food value of 10 hekto-nem, might include:

	Food value (hektonem)
Two large cups of coffee with milk	
200 gm. of water with coffee	0
200 gm. of milk	2
Two lumps of sugar in each cup	
17 gm. of sugar	1
Two rolls of white bread with butter	
50 gm. of white bread	2
8.5 gm. of butter	1
Bacon and eggs	
80 gm. of eggs (2 eggs)	2
20 gm. of bacon (2 small slices)	2
	10

Another example shows the food value of gruel prepared for a child's supper:

260 gm. of milk	260 nem
16 gm. of oatmeal (5 × 16)	80
10 gm. of sugar (10 × 6)	60
	400 nem or 4 Hn.

Von Pirquet insisted not only that the food have adequate nutritive value, but that it should taste good and be appetizing. At his instigation a great many tasty 1-Kn. recipes were worked out in the diet kitchen of the *Kinderklinik*, with explicit directions for their preparation. The amount of seasoning, such as salt, pepper, or onion, was included in the recipe but the slight nutritive values were disregarded.

In a daily diet it is necessary to consider the combustible content of the food, the protein and water content, the vitamins and salts, and the cellulose and other indigestible substances. Physiologists were accustomed to calculate the amount of protein used in metabolism and then arrive at the nitrogen balance. Von Pirquet's approach, however, was to find the natural protein intake, as shown by actual habits at different ages, in different countries, and in different animals. He did not differentiate proteins of varying biological value, but assumed that the supply of essential amino acids in a varied diet was satisfactory. Nor did he try to reach absolute figures for grams of protein per day or per kilogram, but rather he considered the protein used in relation to the amount of combustible material. Humans and domestic animals, regardless of age, apparently take at least 10 per cent—but rarely more than 20 per cent—of their calories in the form of protein. His reasoning was:

Human milk contains about 10 per cent. and bovine milk about 20 per cent. of protein, and we are safe if we keep within these two limits. A less amount may hamper growth and digestion—growth, because proteins are among the most important substances for the body, and digestion, since the different juices of the gastric intestinal tract need proteins to be effective. If sheep, for instance, are fed with too little protein, they are not able to digest starch. On the other hand, a surplus of protein is not used as a structural element, but as a combustible, and it is a very bad one, for a part of it leaves the body through the urine unburnt.

The amount of protein contained in the different food-stuffs is also brought in relation to their value in nem. If 10 per cent. of the food value is contained in the form of protein, we may as well say 1 dekanem (Dn.) of protein is contained in every hektonem of this diet. . . .

The foods listed earlier contain the following amounts of protein:

	Dn. protein in 1 Hn.
Pure fat, oil, butter	0
Sugar, syrup, honey	0
Bacon	0.5
Potatoes	0.5
Fresh fruit	0.5
Flour, biscuit, rice, bread	1
Human milk	1
Fresh fat meat	2
Cow's milk	2
Green peas, turnips, cabbage, cauliflower, lettuce, cucumber	2
Ham, eggs	3
Mushrooms	3
Cheese, skimmed cow's milk	4
Fresh medium meat	4

Thus to determine the amount of protein contained in the breakfast suggested for an adult:

	Dn. protein
2 hektonem of cow's milk (2 Dn. in a Hn.) 2 × 2	4
1 hektonem of sugar	0
2 hektonem of white bread, 1 Dn.	2
1 hektonem of butter	0
2 hektonem of eggs, 3 Dn.	6
2 hektonem of bacon, 0.5	1
	13

Since the 10 hektonem of food in this breakfast contained 13 dekanem of protein, 13 per cent of combustible material was in the form of protein, a figure within the desired range. Von Pirquet did not suggest that the amount of protein be calculated for each meal, but only on a weekly basis. Each week milk, potato, and green vegetables were included to supply vitamins. For all but infants he insisted upon a daily intake of cellulose material—green vegetables or salad at one meal and dark bread twice a day. As fluid he included both that taken directly and the fluid content of solid food. Because water output equals about 95 per cent of an average diet, von Pirquet considered the entire weight of food as water and compared it with the food value in nem. He made up a 400-nem gruel from 260 gm. of milk, 16 gm. flour, and 10 gm. sugar. The total of 286 gm. was reduced by evaporation to 200 gm. which, containing 400 nem, meant that each gram equaled 2 nem. Such a composition, having twice the nutritive value of milk, he called a double-strength food.

He usually recommended that fats, such as butter, lard, or oil, form 10 to 20 per cent of a diet, although he saw no danger in smaller amounts. His views on substitution of fats constituted one of the more controversial aspects of the system.

The fats, as far as they are used as combustibles, can be fully substituted by carbohydrates. The small amount of fat necessary to convey the fat-soluble vitamins can, to my mind, be disregarded in practical feeding in normal times when you are able to give a mixed diet. I have been misunderstood often in my views regarding fat. I never advocated a diet free from fats, but only that a substitution was possible if the conditions of the market made it necessary. At the beginning of the war we had in Austria–Hungary, as a sugar exporting country, a surplus of beet sugar, and, as we were a fat importing country, we soon grew short of fats. We had, therefore, to make the best of the sugar, and I can show that children were able to consume large amounts of sugar as a part of their diet without getting loose bowels or toothache. One has, when giving a large amount of sugar, to be careful to give enough protein in the form of meats, cheese, or milk.

By comparing the spontaneous intake of a great many individuals over long periods of time with their nutritional surface as expressed by the square of the sitting height, von Pirquet determined how many decinem were ingested per square centimeter of absorbing surface or, briefly, the number of "decinem siqua." The square of the sitting height is called *siqua*. As an example, a child whose sitting height is 50 cm. takes 1,250 nem daily. This intake equals 5 decinem multiplied by siqua, or 5 decinem siqua.

The body weight was recorded daily to determine whether the food intake was sufficient. Von Pirquet did not use arithmetical averages, but calculated the mean value graphically. He stated: "We registered a point weekly that corresponded to the change in weight (abscissa) and to the average daily intake for the week in decinem siqua (ordinate). Having registered the records of a large number of children, a graph was constructed by drawing the axis of symmetry through the field of all the points recorded."

The experimental results led to a few practical rules. Four standards for quantitative feeding—the maximum, the minimum, the aequum, and the optimum—were defined as follows:

The *maximum* is the quantity of food that a normal human being can digest within twenty-four hours without impairing his health and without overtaxing his alimentary canal. This maximum is about 1 nem or 10 decinem per square centimeter of the square of the sitting height. . . . Most persons left to themselves never attain that limit except in extraordinary circumstances, as, for instance, after several days of fasting. The *minimum* is the combustible amount necessary to keep the human machine going and to maintain the body weight in a condition of no muscular work except that of chewing and digesting. It is the amount that maintains the person in weight if he lies in bed all the time. This amount is required chiefly for the work of the heart and lungs and for that of the large glands (liver, pancreas, etc.). This minimum corresponds to about 3 decinem siqua. The *aequum* is the amount required to maintain weight under a given condition of activity. Thus, approximately 1 decinem siqua more than the minimum is required when a man works at an occupation that is entirely sedentary instead of lying in bed. If he does some walking besides sitting at his desk he needs 2 decinem siqua in addition to the minimum, or 5 decinem siqua altogether. If he exercises vigorously or does manual labor he needs additional food-stuffs; for a very hard worker the aequum may become identical with the maximum, for he then does all the work possible with the intestinal equipment he has. Such a man becomes a machine for work just as does a horse or ox. On a well-organized farm these animals are run at full speed, eating their maximum, and doing just as much work as possible without loss of weight. The *optimum*, finally, is a conception which includes a judgment; it is the amount of food that should be used by a given person. In a case of heart disease this may be identical with the minimum if we desire to keep the patient in bed as quiet as possible and doing as little digestive work as possible. In most normal adults the optimum is identical with the aequum, for our object is simply to maintain the weight under their condition of work. But there are certain fat or thin adults whose weight we desire to change. In such cases the optimum will be 1 or 2 decinem less or 1 or 2 decinem more than the aequum. In children the optimum is practically always larger than the aequum, as we wish them to grow; hence, we add at least 1 decinem siqua to the aequum. The full amount then provides not only for growth in length but also for growth in fat and muscle.

If an eleven-year-old boy with a sitting height of 70 cm. had a nutritional surface or siqua of 4,900 cm. (70 × 70), the maximum amount that he could digest in twenty-four hours would be 10 decinem (1 nem) per square centimeter, or 4,900 nem. The minimum amount, if he were to remain in bed without moving (and for a healthy boy such inactivity would be practically impossible), would be 3 decinem siqua or 1,470 nem (0.3 × 4,900). Merely to maintain his weight would require 3 decinem siqua more than the minimum, or 6 decinem siqua per day. To provide for growth and for gain in fat and muscle an additional decinem siqua would be needed; thus a total of 7 decinem siqua or 3,430 nem (0.7 × 4,900) per day would be required to achieve the optimum.

For best utilization of food, the child had to be fed equal daily amounts at regular intervals. This principle had long been known to dairy farmers. Because infants can consume only small amounts at a time, von Pirquet divided the daily intake for a newborn baby into eight feedings, given at regular intervals throughout the twenty-four hours. The midnight meal was omitted a few days after birth and the 3:00 A.M. feeding was omitted after two weeks. The remaining six feedings were continued at the same three-hour intervals throughout the first year of life.[11] In the second year the feeding at 9:00 P.M. was omitted but the remaining five feedings were continued during childhood—the main meals in the morning, at midday, and in the evening, and a small meal in mid-morning and mid-afternoon. For adults an exact time was considered less important than that an interval of approximately six hours be observed between meals.

Breast feeding or a substitute was begun when the infant was six hours old. For some days the weight was recorded before and

---

[11] An exact schedule has now been replaced by "demand feeding." Babies, particularly in their first three months, cry not only from hunger or pain but also because of the transition from intrauterine to extrauterine life. When held or given a pacifier they usually become quiet. With this practice there is danger of overfeeding and of the mother not getting enough rest. On the other hand, if the baby oversleeps there is a danger of underfeeding. As in other aspects of child rearing, common sense should prevail. A time schedule is only a guide. The psychoanalysts blame strictness in the first year for anorexia in the second, but demand feeding has been practiced for twenty years and children still do not eat well in the second year. Other factors involved are increased activity and change from a more or less vegetative life to one of rapidly advancing mental development.

after feeding; thereafter, if the mother's milk was adequate, only
the number of feedings and the intervals were regulated. Babies
need adequate water, but the volume of food should not be too
great. If a formula contains too much water the baby cannot drink
all of it and food value is lost; if too little water, the metabolism
becomes disordered. For most children he recommended about
1.5 nem in a weight of 1 gm., never exceeding three times the concentration of milk and rarely going below the concentration of
milk. Von Pirquet called a composition having the same combustible value as human milk a single-strength nutriment (nutri-
mentum simplex), designated by *si*. He formed *sibo* to indicate
simplex bovinum. This food, containing 200 nem in 200 gm., is
composed of:

	Grams	Nem
Milk (3.7% fat)	100	100
Cane sugar	17	100
Water	83	0
	200	200

Infants with a tendency to vomit, who needed food in higher
concentration, were given a double-strength nutriment—duplex
bovinum or *dubo:*

	Grams	Nem
Milk	100	100
Sugar	17	100

The 117 gm. were reduced by evaporation to 100 gm. of weight.
Since they were equivalent to 200 nem, each gram contained
2 nem.

More often an intermediate strength, *sesquibo*, was used:

	Grams	Nem
Milk	100	100
Sugar	8.5	50

This preparation, reduced by evaporation to 100 gm., contained
150 nem.

The maximum food allowance was calculated according to the baby's sitting height. For an infant two months old, whose sitting height was 35 cm., the formula would be:

$$\frac{10}{10} \times \text{Siqua } (35 \times 35) = 1,225 \text{ nem}$$

The optimum food allowance was 6 decinem siqua—3 for minimum needs, 1 for body movements, 1 for growth in length, and 1 for weight increase. The whole day's allowance would be 0.6 × 1,225; each of the six feedings would contain one-tenth of 1,225 or approximately 120 nem. Of *sibo* strength the child would take 120 gm. per feeding; of *dubo*, 60 gm.; of *sesquibo*, 90 gm.

Solid foods were introduced in the middle of the first year, beginning with a double-strength gruel of milk, sugar, and flour to replace milk at the noon meal. At nine months the gruel was given at 6:00 P.M. and vegetables were introduced at noon. Von Pirquet explained how mashed potato might be prepared as a single-strength nutriment:

	Nem
40 gm. of mashed potato	50
50 gm. of milk	50
Water sufficient to make 100 gm.	
A little salt to accustom the baby	
to the taste	

From now on every month some new thing is introduced, such as different vegetables, white bread soaked in milk, biscuits, etc. The breast meals are one by one replaced by other feedings in such a way that at twelve months the child is wholly weaned. During the whole second year the education of the child to take different food-stuffs continues. We call this process "the nutrition school." The baby is taught at this very early age to eat small quantities of almost everything appropriate for the child—bread with butter, jam, eggs, and the last thing, at twenty-four months, is a very small quantity of meat.[12]

To avoid the danger of getting too small an amount of "fat-soluble vitamin" the babies during the winter season get a teaspoonful of cod-

[12] The present practice of introducing solid food at a much younger age is considered highly desirable. Milk is no longer believed to be a sufficient source of essential food factors for the older infant. Meat, on the other hand, is considered less important as long as protein is supplied in other foods.

liver oil daily, which is at the same time calculated in the food value of the diet:

1 teaspoonful = 5 grams of oil × nem value of 13⅓, or approximately 65 nem

The babies are exposed as much as possible to sun and open air. We use for that purpose small balconies put in the windows with southern exposure.

The treatment of premature and malnourished infants followed the same principles. Very weak premature infants were fed sixteen times a day, at equal intervals. When nutrition was poor an exact record was kept of stools and of vomiting, since in many cases of apparent malnutrition the infant had vomited a good deal of the daily intake. When the stools were either normal or small in quantity, the vomiting was usually considered to be a nervous habit. Such an infant was given double-strength nutriment or gruel, with additional food. Those with diarrhea received only water for twelve hours; then the minimum feeding was begun,

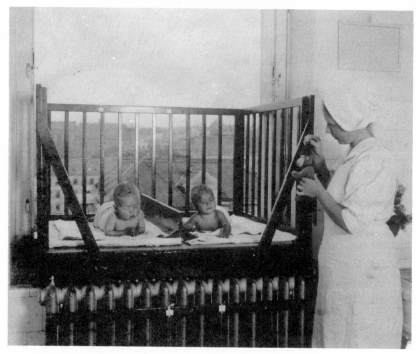

Balcony facing south so that infants could be exposed to sun even in the heart of the city of Vienna.

with small increments until the optimum was resumed. Increasing the energy value of food by preparing it in concentrated form was one of von Pirquet's major contributions to infant nutrition.

Von Pirquet was the undisputed leader of pediatrics in Vienna and it was not long before the successful nutritional results observed in the *Kinderklinik* led others to adopt his system. Almost every section of the city had a children's hospital—a total of fourteen including those privately sponsored—and the method of calculating nutritional requirements from the square of the sitting height was applied in many of them. Portions of the system are still used in the *Kinderklinik*. It was never adopted in the United States.

That the system of nutrition appeared during the early years of the war was not the result, as might be surmised, of governmental attention to economic utilization of food. On the contrary, in an attempt to create an attitude of optimism among the civilian population, official bulletins foretold an early victory which belied the need for conservation. The resultant sense of security diminished rapidly as the war progressed. The armies required a high per capita food ration while at the same time food production in the country was curtailed by a shortage of manpower. Those who did raise crops kept much of the small supply for their own use; imports formerly relied on were entirely cut off. Meat could be obtained, although at a high cost, but the lack of fat was critical.

Even when all of the available food was being carefully conserved, malnutrition was widespread. Infantile scurvy, which had been rare before the war, was then seen frequently. Estimates were that as many as 90 per cent of the younger children showed some degree of rachitic manifestations. One explanation which has been offered was the lack of fuel. At that time coal supplied the necessary power for the plants which made artificial ice. Because Austria was cut off from her coal supply the farmers could not buy ice to cool the raw milk. To prevent souring they treated the milk either by heat or by the addition of a chemical. In either process, as in pasteurization, the vitamin C was destroyed. Ascorbic acid had not yet been discovered, and importation of oranges from Italy was prohibited although, ironically, Italian perfumes could be imported during the postwar period. Children who drank cow's milk were given vitamin C in the form of the juice of Swedish turnips (brassica). Breast-fed infants were thought to be protected from vitamin depletion.

Informed members of the medical profession urged that official action be taken to alleviate the suffering, but needs of the fighting forces received first consideration and little was done to help the general public. Von Pirquet meanwhile worked out the final details of his nutritional method. In America, too, plans were being laid to relieve the starvation in Europe, and as soon as hostilities ceased the American Relief Administration was organized under the direction of Herbert Hoover. Von Pirquet was appointed by the Austrian government as Commissioner General for that country and in May, 1919, working with Hoover, he had the long-awaited opportunity to see his system of nutrition widely applied. The large-scale operation has been described as follows:

The American food is landed at Hamburg, and shipped overland, duty free, to Vienna for the Austrian district. There it is stored in a central warehouse (a wing of the old imperial palace), and distributed on requisition to the district kitchens. These kitchens, often fitted up with old army supplies, cook food for a number of dining rooms in their respective districts. A charming part of the system is that there is no waste. Each dining room supervisor requisitions exactly the number of grams and "nem" prescribed in total for her children; it is delivered hot, about 11 A.M., and the feeding begins at 12.

The children file in, and each presents a card indicating the result of a previous physical examination and the number of "nem" prescribed for him. Serving ladles are standardized in size and so labeled that it becomes an easy matter to dispense any given number of "nem" of food. Each child brings his own container and spoon. This is required in order to prevent cross infection as well as to eliminate dishwashing. After his ration is given him, the child sits at a table and eats his meal. He may stay in the dining room as long as he desires, but he is not permitted to leave the room until his plate is emptied. This rule is insisted on and unless a child is obviously ill, he is compelled to eat his entire prescribed ration. This eliminates the appetite as the index of nutritional needs. It so works out that little trouble is experienced in this respect. The "psychology of the crowd," so dominant in youth, enters and solves the problem, much to the benefit of the child. At stated intervals the children are reexamined, and as soon as their nutritional index reaches a desirable point (at present 94 per cent. "pelidisi"), the child is discharged from the class and a less fortunate individual substituted. . . .

In Austria alone, a maximum of 300,000 children were fed daily, and nearly 1,500,000 children in central Europe ultimately received rations from this source. The governments of the various countries wherein feeding is carried on were anxious to cooperate. The Austrian government, for example, gives the commodities that the country is able to produce, such as flour and vegetables, and it also provides the machinery for the distribution. The American Relief Administration gives such food as the countries in question cannot produce and are too poor to buy (sugar, cocoa, milk, fats and the like). So it actually works out that about two thirds of the cost of feeding is defrayed by the recipient government, and one third by the American Relief Administration. Even so, the American Relief gets a great deal more than one third of the credit. The spontaneous outbursts of gratitude to America evinced by the Austrians, in particular, are the source of much comment by continental visitors.[13]

To provide hundreds of thousands of starving children with even one meal a day was a tremendous task. Its successful accomplishment, due largely to von Pirquet's skillful organization, placed him in an advantageous position to advance some of his ideas on social reform. He emphasized the responsibility of the state for the nutritional welfare of its citizens—a responsibility which had been sadly mishandled during the recent war—and contrasted this failure in the science of nutrition with the marked success in hygiene: "All states have won the war against epidemics; unfortunately this cannot be said about the fight against malnutrition." His humanitarian concepts were heeded and led to enactment of a program directed by the Ministry of Public Health for feeding Austrian school children.

In spite of its complexity, the system of nutrition has been described in detail because it is not well known in the Anglo-Saxon countries and may interest students of the history of medicine and others who are attracted by its practical approach. Some of the characteristics and weaknesses of the system will be considered objectively in the next chapter.

[13] W. E. Carter, "The Pirquet System of Nutrition and Its Applicability to American Conditions," *J. Amer. Med. Assn.* 77 (1921): 1541. (Courtesy of American Medical Association, publisher, Chicago.)

X

Reactions to the Pirquet
System of Nutrition

The popular approval accorded the experiments in nutrition was not generally reflected in medical circles. There, von Pirquet's concepts raised a storm of protest. Certain reviewers ridiculed the system, particularly because of its unfamiliar nomenclature. Von Pirquet was considered an intruder in the field, and it is natural that physiologists and nutritional experts were opposed. Criticism and controversy were strongest in Germany, where the system was never accepted. In spite of hostility, however, it was in Germany that the system of nutrition was first subjected to an unbiased clinical evaluation. Two of the country's leading pediatricians, Edelstein and Langstein, were sufficiently impressed with the successful feeding experiments which had been conducted in Austria to go to the *Kinderklinik* and learn how the nem system operated in a hospital. These two physicians had charge of a famous hospital for infants and preschool children in Berlin, which specialized in nutritional disorders, and there, in 1919, they set aside an entire ward where twenty-four infants were fed according to von Pirquet's method.

The infants in the test group received a regular diet except that the quantity of food was estimated according to their sitting height. Since their diets consisted essentially of milk formulas, conversion from calories to nem was simple. Thirteen of the twenty-four children were less than six months old; six were between six and eight months of age. The number was small, but Edelstein and Langstein were more concerned with testing the practicality of the system through a continuous study of the same children than in collecting abundant clinical data. Other food which the study group received, such as vegetables, gruel, and cereals in milk, was prepared in the same concentration as milk, twice as concentrated, and so forth, and was the same as that given to the entire hospital population. The milk laboratory had been ordered to deliver only the specified proportions during the test period. Almost all infants received 5 decinem per square centimeter of sitting height per day; a few received 6 or 7 decinem later, when they could stand or walk. The only exceptions were that certain children who did not gain weight were given 1 decinem more, usually without success. The formulas were either half milk and half cane sugar of the same concentration as whole milk, varied for some by diluting with a 2 per cent decoction of flour instead of water (equal parts of a milk-flour-cane sugar formula of equal concentration), or a 3:2 concentration, i.e., whole milk with 8.5 per cent cane sugar.

Technical management of the ward and the milk laboratory proved simple as soon as the passive resistance to innovation had been overcome. After the nurses realized the advantage of scooping out food containing the necessary nem with a standard ladle rather than weighing the portions, they acknowledged the ease of preparation.

Young infants tolerated the high sugar and also the disproportionately high protein content. The number and quality of bowel movements were normal with few exceptions. For constipation, half of the sugar was replaced by malt. The cereals prepared with milk and sugar were taken with so much pleasure that they were adopted as part of the routine hospital diet. The experiment was successful except for minor nutritional disturbances. In general, the children thrived, weight gain was satisfactory, and they were resistant to infection. Only two untoward episodes occurred during the period of observation. In one, a three-month-old infant on a formula of whole milk with 8.5 per cent cane sugar, an acute nutritional disorder developed and recovery was slow. This case demonstrated that whole milk is not always safe for young infants[1] and also raised the question of their tolerance for high sugar concentration. The study confirmed that healthy children who are given adequate nursing care can accommodate themselves to various diets.

After analyzing the results of their six-month study, Edelstein and Langstein tried to describe the system impartially at a special meeting of the *Berliner medizinische Gesellschaft* on June 30, 1920, before a somewhat unfriendly audience. They pointed out

---

[1] Today many infants are given undiluted whole milk, or evaporated milk brought to whole-milk strength by the addition of water, without subsequent discomfort. Of course, the sterility of the milk is now more rigidly controlled.

that von Pirquet's system justified careful scrutiny even though it raised doubts about Rubner's theory and caloric measurements. Their experiments led to the conclusion that certain controversial details, such as nomenclature, should not cause the entire nem system to be rejected but that criticism should be restricted to three points.

1. *Calculation of nutritional requirements from intake of food instead of from loss of heat.*

No objection was raised to the logic of determining nutritional requirements from intake of food or of basing calculations on the nutritional surface. They did wonder why von Pirquet preferred to make derivations from the two-thirds power of ten times the body weight. However, whereas he considered hunger and complete rest to be exceptional states, they felt that Rubner's rest and fasting values provided insight into the basal metabolic rate from which, with the addition of experiments after ingestion of food and after exercise, all other measurements could be ascertained. They quoted other workers to demonstrate that values calculated from heat loss were not purely experimental, as von Pirquet had suggested.

They pointed out that a workingman eats to maintain his basal metabolism, not his normal body temperature. This, like any other arbitrary turnover of energy, is calculated from the balance of energy; i.e., the production of heat is calculated by measuring heat loss. They considered von Pirquet's method no more accurate than that hitherto prevailing, especially since he himself had admitted that the standard applied to these calculations was arbitrary.

2. *Replacement of the calorie by another unit.*

Edelstein and Langstein defined the calorie as not just a physical or chemical unit but as a physiological measure entirely suited for hospital use. Rubner's standard values were based upon a varied normal diet, not on pure foodstuffs. A calorimetric survey of the human on a varied diet, either at rest or exercising, showed excellent agreement between calculated and observed values. Furthermore, the caloric determination correlated with other physical units. They believed that by converting calories into nem, von Pirquet had slightly overestimated the protein minimum of human milk. In this oversimplification a generation of students taught only the use of milk units might lose sight of important correlations with the science of nutrition. The endless confusion of large and small, crude and utilizable calories was considered unjustified when tables showing the utilization of foodstuffs were available. Nevertheless, the von Pirquet system was superior in its easy comparison of prepared dishes with an equivalent concentration of milk. Another advantage of the nem system was the simple relation of the nutritional unit to the surface unit—that is, of 1 gm. of milk to 1 sq. cm. of intestinal surface—although they doubted that the entire intestinal surface had uniform resorptive power. Milk units calculated from the square of the sitting height yielded uniform results with a freely chosen amount of food.

3. *Von Pirquet's quantitative concept, particularly his view that fat could be entirely replaced by carbohydrates.*

Here the criticism was directed toward von Pirquet's overemphasis of energetic, isodynamic considerations at the expense of the qualitative principle. In his contention that fat could be replaced by calorically equivalent amounts of carbohydrate, they felt he had been influenced by the successful experiments in fattening cattle on fodder low in fat. When he went so far as to withhold fat from the growing infant, they questioned some of his results.

As early as 1918, several investigators had warned against equicaloric exchange because of breeding failures in rats given a fat-free diet, and stressed that some fats could take up the vitamins which were essential for normal growth. Even von Gröer, von Pirquet's coworker, had had questionable success in his attempts to support von Pirquet's concept by prolonged experiments on infants. Similarly, animal experiments and new methods of feeding children, undertaken by Anglo-Saxon investigators, demonstrated that an equicaloric exchange of fat and carbohydrate was unsatisfactory because different amounts of fat-soluble vitamins were present in the fats.[2]

Fats, like all other foodstuffs, are split in the intestinal canal. In contrast to the proteins, however, they can be rebuilt immedi-

[2] F. Edelstein, and L. Langstein, "Das Pirquet'sche System der Ernährung," *Berlin. klin. Wchnschr.* 57 (part 2) (1920): 823, 852.

ately in the intestinal wall and stored as a fat reserve. Significant here is the contrast between ingested fat and stored fat. One component of fat, glycerin, which the organism itself can synthesize, remains fairly constant, but the fatty-acid radicals may vary a great deal. In regard to the capability of the cell to produce synthetic components of the fatty acids, our knowledge is still rather obscure. It is possible that a disturbance in the intermediary metabolism may be precipitated either by inability of the cell to produce certain components of the fat, if the organism is depending upon its own body fat, or by fat formed synthetically from carbohydrate, as happens with fat-free nutrition. The cell may either effect synthesis of a somewhat different type, or available split products may be withdrawn from their proper function and diverted to exactly this performance. In either circumstance, damage results. One can even imagine cases in which the organism must produce fats in a more solid or a more liquid state, as protection against exterior or interior changes. The turnover of energy always remains essentially the same; the qualitatively material process will take a different course each time. These and other considerations, such as the danger of overloading the intestinal tract with excess carbohydrate or the importance of vitamins, left von Pirquet's theory open to discussion. Although the fat problem is not an integral constituent of his system, it demonstrates the conclusions to which a one-sided emphasis on the quantitative principle may lead.

In accord with contemporary thinking, von Pirquet classified foodstuffs as building materials or fuel; by and large, this classification is correct but its emphasis on energy metabolism may be highly dangerous, particularly during childhood when both the rate of body growth and the quality of the increment are important. No living matter grows without a source of energy, yet even a good supply of energy will not produce growth in a state of chemical imbalance.

Edelstein and Langstein's lecture was followed by a heated discussion, and opinion was divided. Some thought replacement of the calorie by the nem was unnecessary, others that it was easier for the layman to understand. Some contended that milk was not a truly physiological unit, others that the idea of calculating body surface from the square of the sitting height was not original with von Pirquet. The strongest rejection came from

Czerny, von Pirquet's old antagonist, who denied that the system had any scientific justification and criticized the nomenclature as needlessly complicated. Even a decade later, in an obituary, Czerny was critical. He praised von Pirquet's early work as the lasting product of a superior mind, but stated that the contributions of later years did not merit commendation and that the complicated nutritional system would not survive. As an authority in the field of nutrition, Pfaundler was asked for an opinion. He did not enter the controversy, although he did state that the calorie must remain the common standard. Like Edelstein and Langstein, many other pediatricians who had applied the nem system in their hospitals reacted quite favorably.

Infant nutrition presented serious problems in the early years of the twentieth century and infant mortality was high. Pediatricians did not know the role of enzymes in digestion, nor that disease was produced by ingested pathogens and not by the bacteria normally present in the intestine. Nutritional disorders were variously interpreted, and the individual components of milk were blamed when an infant failed to thrive. Milk powders and evaporated milk were unknown, and artificial feeding was considered risky. Mechanical refrigerators did not exist and even the old-fashioned icebox was not found in the average low-income household. Most infants were breast fed. Special formulas for the sick were too complicated to be prepared at home and were not available commercially. As a result, all sorts of "curative formulas" were recommended, and theories and procedures came and went like fads. Frustrating attempts to approximate the chemical structure of cow's milk and breast milk dominated pediatric thinking. Von Pirquet simplified infant feeding by doing away with the complicated formulas and making no attempt to adjust the chemical composition of cow's milk. For him breast feeding was still a *noli me tangere*. One may avoid a slavish imitation of breast milk and yet adhere to its chemical constitution, but this von Pirquet was not inclined to do. He did compensate for the disturbance in ion equilibrium due to the dilution of cow's milk by adding 45 per cent potassium glycerophosphate, approximately 80 per cent potassium chloride, and a trace of iron, but he estimated the ash, the fat, and the dry matter mainly in terms of nem. In his *Klinik* the infant formulas consisted only of milk, water, and granulated cane sugar. This is similar to the present practice with the exception that solid food is now introduced earlier in the first year of life.

The greatest progress in infant nutrition came with the introduction of bacteriologically safe pasteurized milk and milk products, introduction of accessory foods during the first year of life, and the education of mothers in proper techniques of feeding. The belief that breast milk was superior to cow's milk is no longer held, and retrospectively it appears as though a virtue had been made of necessity. Nevertheless, the possibility of the transfer of antibodies through breast milk cannot be denied. Progress also came with an understanding of the metabolic changes which accompany nutritional disorders, particularly derangement of the electrolyte balance in sick children, and treatment by the intravenous route. In von Pirquet's time this concept had not developed, and intravenous treatment was just beginning. But he introduced strict quantitative principles and abandoned the artificial theories of his contemporaries.

A revised edition of a widely circulated textbook on nutritional disturbances of the infant was published near the end of von Pirquet's life. The concepts expressed in the new edition were entirely unlike those in his own system of nutrition and he considered some of them quite artificial. He commented that the devices which had been used to substantiate the author's hypotheses reminded him of Ptolemaic attempts, after Galileo had in-invented the telescope, to refute the Copernican system of astronomy and to justify the ancient beliefs on the basis of epicycles. The theory of epicycles, it will be remembered, was used to explain the orbits of the planets according to a geocentric *Weltanschauung*, or philosophy of life.

In spite of the attacks, von Pirquet adhered firmly to his convictions. He did not retract what he considered to be his contribution to the science of nutrition, particularly infant feeding. He believed one reason for its lack of acceptance was that his nutritional system employed an unfamiliar unit.

More friendly than the German response were comments from the United States and England. One of the two important American articles was written by William E. Carter:

Most of the criticisms in America of this system are leveled at the fact that the calorie, which is well established in this country as the unit of feeding, is replaced by the "nem." It is unfortunate that the term "nem system" is used in describing it, as the "nem" is the least part of the philosophy. The term "Pirquet system" is a far better one, as it epitomizes all the essential facts—the nutritional estimations as well as the feeding methods. The system includes a host of details, singular in their simplicity, yet representing all the accepted principles of nutrition, based on strict mathematical formulas. . . .

We believe that the Pirquet system is applicable to American conditions, especially those under which it may be desirable to feed children in considerable numbers. The method appeals to us for the following reasons:

It provides a simple, accurate and rapid method of estimating the nutritional status easily grasped by workers even without medical training, and it impresses them in a graphic way with the necessity of proper nutrition; it reduces the prescribing of the requisite food intake to a simple formula based on the sitting height as a constant; it makes it possible by the use of a single word to make a record of the child's nutritional state which may serve for comparison with the results of future examinations; it eliminates waste and at the same time it provides the child with an adequate amount of food to cover his needs and, by its very operation, it insures the actual ingestion of the food; it serves as a selective agent, at once segregating children into various groups— those with moderate need, those with urgent need and those without need of additional food. . . .

The experience of Mr. Hoover and Professor Pirquet in central Europe is ample evidence that the nutritional status of children fed by this method is markedly improved in a surprisingly short time. The sending of food for the relief of the children of central Europe was highly commendable; in fact, it was one of the most generous things that history records. Yet we should not overlook the fact that many of our own children, judged by the same standards employed by the American Relief Administration, are in need of supplemental food.[3]

Other favorable comments were directed by Faber to American pediatricians:

Of the many innovations and ingenuities for which the war was responsible, none are more interesting than those which were devised and forced into practice in the attempt adequately to feed the peoples of belligerent countries on a reduced food supply. There have recently come to this country some accounts of the system of feeding, intended primarily for children in institutions but later given a much wider

[3] W. E. Carter, "The Pirquet System of Nutrition and Its Applicability to American Conditions," *J. Amer. Med. Assn.* 77 (1921): 1541. (Courtesy of American Medical Association, publisher, Chicago.)

application, which von Pirquet introduced in Vienna early in the war. Von Pirquet has published a book expounding the system, which is not yet available here. . . . The system possesses much matter of interest to students of nutrition as an ingenious and novel attempt to rearrange the data of nutritional science with the purpose of obtaining popular interest and comprehension for scientific feeding, and of making the fullest possible utilization of available foods while obtaining for each individual his just quota of food and eliminating waste. To these ends a thorough-going reform of current practice in feeding was attempted not only in institutions but in the home, in restaurants, in community kitchens and, indeed, wherever groups of people were fed. . . .

Von Pirquet's objection to the use of the calorie as the unit of food value lay largely in the considerations of popular psychology. His idea was that the conception of food units as heat units is so abstract that not only the laity but most professional men as well fail to connect it with reality and for practical purposes search for a more direct means of comparison. Many physicians, for instance, compare foods with the egg as a unit of value. Von Pirquet believed that a direct comparison unit of this sort would win general acceptance by its direct imaginative appeal. Thus the first step in popular education in the scientific use of food would be gained. Milk, as the first and only specifically physiological food, was selected as his standard of comparison.[4]

The *British Medical Journal,* in a review of Mayerhofer and von Pirquet's textbook on nutrition,[5] stated that the system was "a brilliant success in practice" and continued:

The nem system in its most perfect expression can be studied best in the University Kinderklinik in Vienna, of which Professor Pirquet is the director. Here the entire diets of all the children are controlled in this way. A large ward of convalescent tuberculous children between the ages of 6 and 14, who lead a moderately normal life, is the most interesting example. The kitchens of the hospital, including the "milk kitchen" where the food of all infants is prepared, are presided over by expert sisters; all cooking is done on strict quantitative lines, so that the exact composition and calorie value of every cooked dish are accurately known. These kitchens serve as schools for teaching this branch of the nem system. . . .[6]

Even the most benevolent critics interpreted the system of nutrition as a product of the postwar starvation in Central

[4] H. K. Faber, "Von Pirquet's Feeding System," *Amer. J. Dis. Child.* 19 (1920): 478.
[5] *Lehrbuch der Volksernährung nach dem Pirquet'schen System* (Vienna: Urban and Schwarzenberg, 1920). (With E. Mayerhofer.)
[6] "Review. The 'Nem' System of Nutrition," *Brit. Med. J.* 2 (1920): 666.

Europe. Actually, it originated in a period when economic need did not exist. During the favorable economy before World War I, food was in such plentiful supply that selection depended upon individual preference. The inferior fats and cereals which lacked taste appeal were sold so cheaply that real hunger occurred in a negligible percentage of the population. During the war emergency the quantity of food was reduced to such an extent that free purchase and subjective satiation had to be replaced by a per capita allotment which would provide adequate food to keep each citizen alive and able to accomplish his assigned tasks. To meet these needs von Pirquet drew on two existing resources—his standard for the nutritional value of food and a new criterion for the nutritional requirements of the individual.[7]

His ideas on the importance of nutrition in preventive medicine developed rather early. At that time exact nutritional requirements received consideration only in the milk laboratory of a children's hospital. After infancy, little attention was paid to individual requirements. He was the first to suggest the separate role of the hospital dietitian and the nurse, a change not generally adopted until much later. He emphasized that the cook, like the pharmacist, should receive scientific training so that she might perform her work accurately and with clear understanding: "It is an easy thing to teach the fundamental principles about food values and all that, but the chief problem is to make a cook or a grandmother believe in the practice of scientific feeding. It is one thing to prescribe a medicine and another thing to prepare it. We may have some idea how a prescription should be compounded, but most of us would be lost without a pharmacist to do it." The Austrian nurses looked upon cooking as an art, but considered it greatly inferior to nursing. Von Pirquet tried to make them realize the significance of nutrition by declaring that the kitchen was more important than the pharmacy. When he assigned his best nurses to supervise the kitchen, he obtained excellent co-operation. In order to make nutrition "so effective that real statistical results can be obtained we cannot be satisfied if proper feeding principles be applied to individuals or to a small

[7] Sitzung der Berliner mediz. Gesellschaft zu Ehren der Vereinigten Aerztlichen Abteilungen der Waffenbrüderlichen Vereinigungen (Session of the Berlin Medical Society in honor of the United Medical Divisions of the Unions of Comrades in Arms), 1918.

group of people. We must try to make the science of nutrition a part of the education of the people at large."[8]

It is not easy to evaluate the system of nutrition, but no serious critique can neglect the abundance of ingenious and fundamentally new thoughts. After a thorough study of the system, one is impressed by its simplicity of design. On the other hand, those with less understanding can be confused by some of the details. Von Pirquet intended to draw a simple plan with a few short lines, but under his hands an edifice—artistic, indeed, but rather complicated—developed. His anthropometric studies, particularly the fundamental relation of body weight to nutritional surface, are of lasting value, but the nomenclature placed a burden on the system which discouraged many at the outset. The introduction of formulas having caloric equivalence to various volumes of whole milk is ingenious and important. No less important are the economic and sociopolitical possibilities of controlling the nutrition of large populations by a simple procedure.

Contemporaries are not always the most competent judges. It is innate in human nature to degrade and belittle innovations, particularly if they come from an outsider, and such von Pirquet was in the science of nutrition. Little wonder that he sometimes met pungent opposition and criticism. In his maturity he abstained from responding to the "uproar on the street" and left the judgment to posterity. A half-century later we can evaluate the system of nutrition more dispassionately from the viewpoint of *its specific structure, its origin, the peculiarities of its nomenclature, and its ideological background.* Now we realize that the controversy was not always based on scientific reasoning but stemmed from more personal motives. The old antithesis between genius and talent leads to conflict if talent fails to understand intuition.

[8] *An Outline of the Pirquet System of Nutrition* (Philadelphia: W. B. Saunders Co., 1922).

XI

The Last Period

In the third and last of his creative periods, which occurred during the postwar era, most of von Pirquet's scientific interest centered in the field of biostatistics. His mind indulged in abstractions and he was fascinated by numbers and graphic analyses. His intellectual satisfaction may be compared to that of a music lover enjoying a Bach fugue. It was no longer *what* he conceived that was of importance to him, but *the way* it was expressed and exhibited. The construction and arrangement of charts reached a degree of artistic perfection which was characteristic of his activity during that time. A detailed discussion of the work of this period, which culminated in what he termed allergy of the life phases, would in itself require a complete monograph because of the many charts and tables essential to its full understanding, but a study of selected incidents will demonstrate where his attention was chiefly directed.

In spite of a certain antagonism toward the man of genius, and individual differences of opinion which are the inevitable reaction to those who blaze new frontiers, von Pirquet was highly esteemed in Germany. His tenure as professor of pediatrics in Breslau had been short, yet his reputation there was such that a great many students from the Reich studied in Vienna for a *Kultursemester* or two. He also attracted German physicians who came to his clinic for postgraduate training in pediatrics. A young German pediatrician who was one of his great admirers was Rudolf Degkwitz of Munich, who introduced convalescent serum for prophylaxis against measles. Degkwitz liked to discuss his problems with von Pirquet, and was a welcome guest in Vienna.

In the 1920's the two major centers of pediatrics in Germany were Munich and Berlin. In each university the chair of pediatrics was occupied by an Austrian—that in Munich by Pfaundler, in Berlin by Czerny. Pfaundler had a subtle and scholarly mind. He and von Pirquet had much in common, and the two were always on the best of terms. Czerny was of entirely different stature and disposition. He had succeeded Heubner, whose pioneering activity in German pediatrics was comparable to that of Emmett Holt in the United States. Von Pirquet had studied under Heubner, always held him in high esteem, and displayed his picture. The same rapport did not exist with Czerny, and tension between them was often obvious. On one occasion when he was in Vienna, Czerny visited the *Kinderklinik* and was invited to attend von Pirquet's rounds. When the group reached the infants' ward, Czerny inquired about a diagnosis and was handed the chart on which the patient's daily record, including all intake and output, had been plotted. Great care was taken in the preparation of these charts, which permitted the physician to note the findings at a glance instead of reading a lengthy description. Czerny brushed the chart aside with the comment that he did not care much for it. At this tactless remark, von Pirquet left the ward and his assistants continued the rounds. The subject was not mentioned when he and Czerny met again after rounds had been concluded.

Czerny's field was nutrition and, as mentioned earlier, he disagreed violently with the nem system. The Czerny–Keller textbook on nutritional disorders of infancy[1] was recognized as authoritative in its time, yet little of the thinking has survived. On the other hand, most of von Pirquet's views on infant feeding, which were remarkably simple for an era when pasteurized milk was not generally used and nutritional fads were rampant, are still valid.

Heubner's close personal knowledge of the two men led him to make a remark which must be considered a classic appraisal. He compared von Pirquet's brain with a gold balance, Czerny's with a weighbridge. The aptness of this simile is illustrated by von Pirquet's study of the seasonal distribution of fatal illnesses. He presented what he called the center of gravity of disease, a concept unique, ingenious, and appropriate for his gold-balance brain, assembling the data in the form of an astronomical map. This article is difficult to understand. There is little text and the theory is explained chiefly through graphics and equations.

The mortality figures on which the study was based were those recorded by the Office of the Registrar General for England and

---

[1] A. D. Czerny, and A. Keller, *Des Kindes Ernährung, Ernährungsstörungen und Ernährungstherapie* (Vienna: Franz Deuticke, 1925).

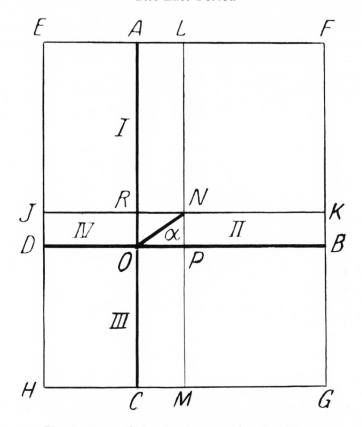

Fig. 18. Diagram for locating the center of gravity. The two lines of gravity intersect at *N. From:* "Die Todeskrankheiten in ihrer jahreszeitlichen Verteilung," *Ztschr. f. Kinderheilk.* 44 (1927): 413. (Courtesy of Springer-Verlag, Heidelberg.)

Wales[2] for 1912 to 1920. From tables showing deaths in the four quarters of each year, von Pirquet determined by trigonometric calculation the center of gravity, or day with highest frequency of fatalities, for each illness.

According to a co-ordinate system, deaths occurring in the first quarter of the year were registered on the positive ordinate *OA* (line I), those in the second quarter on the positive abscissa *OB* (line II), those in the third quarter on the negative ordinate *OC* (line III), and those in the fourth quarter on the negative abscissa *OD* (line IV) (Fig. 18). A rectangle (*EFGH*) was con-

---

[2] Their mortality statistics were the oldest in the world, dating from 1840, and were von Pirquet's chief source of reliable information.

structed parallel to abscissa and ordinate, its sides being I + III and II + IV. To determine the center of gravity the sides *EH* and *FG* were bisected and line *JK* was drawn to represent one of the lines of gravity. The process was repeated for sides *EF* and *HG* and the other line of gravity *LM* was drawn. The two lines of gravity intersect at *N* which is the center of gravity of the rectangle. The two important pieces of data are (1) the distance of the center of gravity from the center *O*, i.e., the straight line *ON*, and (2) angle α *NOP*. They can be calculated as follows:

$$NP = LP - LN = AO - AR$$

$$AO = \text{I.} \quad AR = \frac{AC}{2} = \frac{AO + OC}{2} = \frac{\text{I} + \text{III}}{2}$$

$$NP = \text{I} - \frac{\text{I} + \text{III}}{2} = \frac{\text{I} - \text{III}}{2}$$

$$OP = OB - PB = \text{II} - \frac{\text{II} + \text{IV}}{2} = \frac{\text{II} - \text{IV}}{2}$$

$$\text{Tangent } \alpha = NP{:}OP = \frac{\text{I} - \text{III}}{2} : \frac{\text{II} - \text{IV}}{2} = \frac{\text{I} - \text{III}}{\text{II} - \text{IV}}$$

$$ON = \sqrt{(NP)^2 + (OP)^2} = \sqrt{\left(\frac{\text{I} - \text{III}}{2}\right)^2 + \left(\frac{\text{II} - \text{IV}}{2}\right)^2}$$

$$= \frac{1}{2}\sqrt{(\text{I} - \text{III})^2 + (\text{II} - \text{IV})^2}.$$

If I – III (difference between fatalities in the first and third quarters) is called *A*, and II – IV (difference between fatalities in the second and fourth quarters) is called *B*,

$$\text{then tangent } \alpha = A/B$$

$$ON = 1/2\sqrt{A^2 + B^2}.$$

By means of angle α one can determine the exact date of the center of gravity. Suppose it is 40 degrees in the schematic diagram (Fig. 18). Each month is considered to have 30 days and the year 360 days to correspond with 360 degrees in a circle; hence each degree represents one day. The positive abscissa on which figures for the second quarter are registered is midway between April 1 and July 1, or May 15. Angle α is calculated back from positive abscissa II by 40 degrees, or 40 days, which places the center of gravity on April 5.

If *NP* were greater than *OP*, the angle would be over 45 degrees and the tangent would be measured for angle

$$NOR: \frac{NR}{OR} \text{ or } \frac{II - IV}{I - III}.$$

A circle with *O* as the center can be divided into octants (Fig. 19). The positive ordinate corresponds to the middle of the first quarter and separates the first from the second octant of the year. The first octant is therefore at the left of the positive ordinate. The angle is situated in the third octant, since *A* was smaller than *B*. If *A* had been greater than *B*, the center of gravity would fall in the second quarter. If both *A* and *B* are positive, the center of gravity will fall in the right upper quadrant; in that case I must

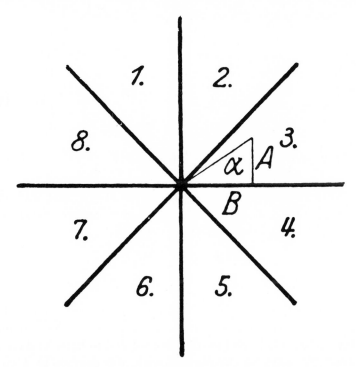

Fig. 19. Shows octants and angle α. *From:* "Die Todeskrankheiten in ihrer jahreszeitlichen Verteilung," *Ztschr. f. Kinderheilk.* 44 (1927): 414. (Courtesy of Springer–Verlag, Heidelberg.)

be greater than III, and II greater than IV. If B is negative (II smaller than IV) and A positive, the center of gravity is in the left upper quadrant. The following table shows the factors upon which the octant depends and how it can be determined from the differences of I − III and II − IV.

| I − III | II − IV | $A − B$ | |
A	B	D	Octant
+	−	+	1
+	+	+	2
+	+	−	3
−	+	−	4
−	+	+	5
−	−	+	6
−	−	−	7
+	−	−	8

This table can be entered into the circle of the year if the beginning of the year is directed toward north and the coordinate system is turned 45 degrees to the right.

Typhoid fever was chosen to illustrate the calculations, and fatalities for both sexes for the quarters from 1912–20[3] were totaled:

First quarter	(I)	2,396
Second quarter	(II)	2,213
Third quarter	(III)	2,259
Fourth quarter	(IV)	2,769
Total		9,637

From figures for A, B, and D von Pirquet calculated the center of gravity.

$$A = (I − III) = 2,396 − 2,259 = +137$$
$$B = (II − IV) = 2,213 − 2,769 = −556$$
$$D = (A − B) = +137 − 556 = −419$$

The eighth octant has been shown to have signs + − −, where angle α has to be added to 315 (Fig. 20). It is calculated from the tangent by dividing the smaller by the greater figure, in this example A (137) by B (556) or 246, which corresponds to an

[3] The period from July 1, 1918, to June 30, 1919, was not included.

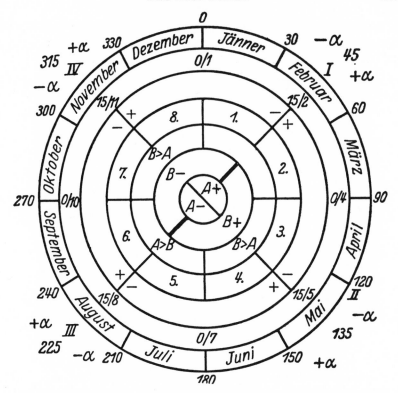

Fig. 20. Auxiliary guide for determining date of center of gravity. *From:* "Die Todeskrankheiten in ihrer jahreszeitlichen Verteilung," *Ztschr. f. Kinderheilk.* 44 (1927): 416. (Courtesy of Springer–Verlag, Heidelberg.)

angle of 14 degrees. The center of gravity is thus 315 + 14 or 329, and occurs on November 29.

Next he determined line *ON* as

$$1/2\sqrt{(I - III)^2 + (II - IV)^2}.$$

Since only the relative length of the lines is of importance, the ½ can be omitted:

$$A\ (137)^2 = 18,700$$
$$B\ (556)^2 = 309,000$$
$$ON = 572$$

This figure represents the preponderance of deaths in a specific quarter of the year. If we assume 100 deaths from a disease, all in the first quarter, *ON* would equal

$$\sqrt{(I - III)^2 + (II - IV)^2} = \sqrt{(100 - 0)^2 + (0 - 0)} = 100$$

If 10,000 persons died from another disease, likewise all in the first quarter, ON would be 10,000. The seasonal incidence of the two diseases would be identical; they would differ only in the absolute number of fatalities, a factor which is not pertinent. To eliminate this factor, the ratio of ON to the absolute number of deaths was established by using it as divisor and multiplying by 1,000. This means that if 1,000 deaths per year occurred from the disease in question, R (radius) would coincide with the maximum point for the year (the center of gravity).

$$R = \frac{\sqrt{(I - III)^2 + (II - IV)^2}}{I + II + III + IV} \times 1,000 = \frac{1,000}{S} \sqrt{A^2 + B^2}$$

In the case of typhoid fever

$$R = \frac{1,000}{S} \sqrt{A^2 + B^2} = \frac{1,000}{9,637} \times 572 = 59.5.$$

From the mortality tables a diagram was constructed (Fig. 21). For each year the center of gravity was calculated but not the radius. The epidemic peak occurs in the winter months and therefore the calendar year was not used. The entire report covered the period from July 1, 1912 to June 30, 1920. Because the influenza pandemic distorted the figures, the year 1918–19 was omitted. Where numbers were large enough, the center of gravity was calculated for each individual year. Here the grouping of illnesses refers to the average center of gravity, including the year 1918 to 1919.

The centers of gravity of all diseases were assembled according to the day of the year and the radius (Fig. 21). Between the outermost circle, corresponding to a radius of 400, and the next circle within (at a radius of 380) each day was represented by a radial line. For the center of gravity of typhoid (enteric) fever the number 330–329 was determined; near the center, at the radius of 60, a cross marks the center of gravity. Epidemiological groupings showed that malignant tumors were almost uninfluenced by the season, in contrast to the acute infections. The pulmonary diseases (February) and acute disorders of the gastrointestinal tract (beginning in September) were strongly seasonal. Tuberculous fatalities occurred particularly from February through May, the respiratory tuberculoses at the beginning of this period,

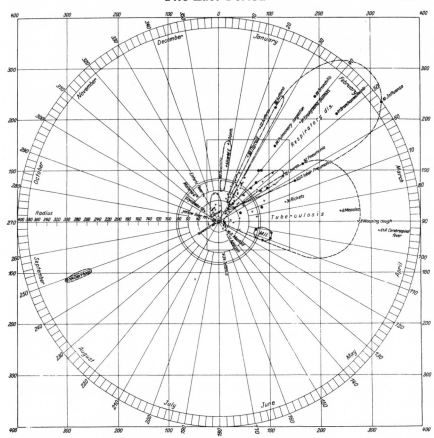

Pirquet, Todeskrankheiten   Schwerpunkte der Todeskrankheiten   Photol. u. Druck v. C. Keller, Berlin

Fig. 21. Centers of gravity of fatal illnesses. *From:* "Die Todeskrankheiten in ihrer jahreszeitlichen Verteilung," *Ztschr. f. Kinderheilk.* 44 (1927). (Courtesy of Springer–Verlag, Heidelberg.)

meningitis and miliary tuberculosis at the end. Late winter was the peak period of deaths from many diseases in the septic-respiratory group.[4]

Von Pirquet was very proud of this accomplishment, as an artist prizes his creation, and prior to publication he read the paper at the 1927 meeting of the *Deutsche Gesellschaft für Kinderheilkunde* in Budapest. In spite of its complexity, the presentation was well received.

---

[4] "Die Todeskrankheiten in ihrer jahreszeitlichen Verteilung," *Ztschr. f. Kinderheilk.* 44 (1927): 413. (Courtesy of Springer–Verlag, Heidelberg.)

Afterward, while sitting at dinner in a restaurant, he was most cheerful and witty. As he studied the menu he whispered into my ear: "The Hungarian menus should list three kinds of meat—boiled, fried, and ridden under the saddle." He was referring to the legend that the horsemen of the Huns tenderized meat by keeping it beneath the saddle while they rode. This implication that the Magyars retained Hunnish blood is not very flattering to the Hungarians; their origin is still debatable. When the meetings of the society were concluded the *Kinderklinik* group returned to Vienna in a small aircraft, our first flying experience. Von Pirquet was still in high spirits and especially enjoyed viewing his estate in Hirschstetten from the air. Nevertheless he was well aware that his entire inner staff, including among them his potential successor, were in a shaky airplane and he remarked what a chance there would be for a new professor of pediatrics in case of accident.

A few years after the war ended, von Pirquet was invited to give a series of medical lectures in the United States. This gesture of friendship was the first such invitation to be issued to an Austrian citizen after the cessation of World War I, and resulted in the Silliman lectures on nutrition at Yale University in the winter of 1921–22 and a Harvey lecture at the New York Academy of Medicine on the importance of nutrition in tuberculosis.

The close working relationship with members of the Rockefeller Foundation during the years immediately after the war had led to a continuing friendship, and when in New York von Pirquet visited the Rockefeller Institute for Medical Research. He told me afterward that while there he was reminded of the story of a Hapsburg emperor of the Middle Ages who reigned at the time the Gothic cathedral of St. Stephen in Vienna, started in the eleventh century, was nearing completion. The emperor wanted St. Stephen's to be known as one of the outstanding cathedrals of all time, but he was aware that this result could not be achieved through architecture alone. To gain real distinction, the cathedral would have to be the site of many miracles. Therefore the emperor gave instructions that the remains of miracle-working saints buried throughout the empire were to be brought together to St. Stephen's. When this order was carried out, the people who had formerly gone to a country church near their homes to ask special help of a favorite saint had to make the long trip to Vienna.

But in the large new cathedral no miracles were performed. Von Pirquet felt that the medical miracle workers similarly lost their power to perform when they were uprooted from the scene of their early accomplishments and moved into the modern setting of the Rockefeller Institute.

It was not long before efforts were begun to bring him back to America on a more permanent basis, this time to St. Paul, Minnesota, where funds were being raised for a new children's hospital. In June, 1923, von Pirquet went to Edinburgh to present a paper to the International Physiological Congress on the relationship of pulse rate to sitting height, and the dean of the University of Minnesota medical faculty arranged to meet him there. Letters had previously been exchanged, and at their meeting the dean offered him the chair of pediatrics, which he agreed to accept. In 1924, when he arrived to take the appointment, he discovered that pediatrics was a new department which he was expected to organize. He was disappointed in the facilities which were available, and too impatient to wait the somewhat indeterminate period of time until construction of the hospital could be undertaken. In a brief mention of this episode Rowntree commented that "Dr. von Pirquet seemed unable to settle down to real work."[5] There is little doubt but that Madame von Pirquet's displeasure with the surroundings was a large factor in precipitating their departure. Von Pirquet was greatly upset by the outcome. He did not stop on the east coast to visit his old friends in New York, at the Johns Hopkins University, or in Philadelphia, presumably because he did not wish to explain the frustrating details. It was his final visit to the United States. Although he left St. Paul hastily, he seemed in no hurry to go home. He traveled to Europe in leisurely fashion on a ship which crossed the Atlantic by the southern route. Even after he returned to Vienna he was reluctant to discuss the episode, and it was some time before he regained his equipoise and appeared to be his former self.

By the 1920's he had become a national figure, and toward the end of the decade he was nominated as a candidate for president of the Austrian Republic. In the early years of the Republic men of prominence were considered for the presidential office rather than politicians. Herbert Hoover was delighted to learn of

[5] L. G. Rowntree, *Amid Masters of Twentieth Century Medicine* (Springfield, Illinois: C. C Thomas, 1958).

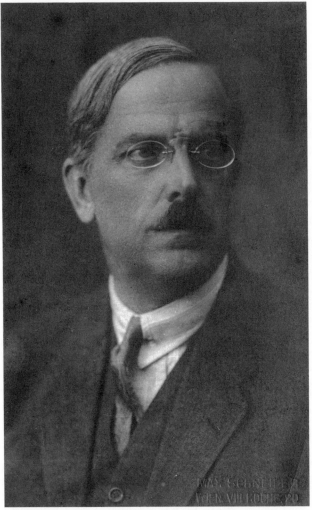

Von Pirquet in 1928. (Photograph by Max Schneider, Vienna.)

this honor and was the first to send a cable of congratulation. Von Pirquet himself was pleased to be offered the opportunity for public service. When I asked him how he expected to deal with the duties of the position he jokingly answered: "I am not worried. I am sure there must be a short and simple directory of procedures for a president as there is for a police officer." This problem did not arise because his name was not chosen to appear on the ballot.

In conjunction with the Rockefeller Foundation, the League of Nations sponsored public health education throughout the world. Courses were held and scientific ideas were exchanged. When an international congress of health officers was held in Vienna in 1923, von Pirquet addressed the group on the subject of pediatric hospitalization in Austria. The idea of establishing a permanent committee to study the problems of child health originated with him. He made the suggestion in a letter to Dr. L. Rajchman, secretary of the Hygiene Section of the League, and recommended that members be selected to represent a language group rather than a nation: for French-speaking countries, Nobécourt; for English, Findlay; for Dutch, Scheltema; for Spanish, Morquio; and for German, himself. The proposal was accepted and the Committee for Child Hygiene was formed, as a subsidiary of the Hygiene Section, with von Pirquet as chairman. Its membership, however, was not limited to the group von Pirquet had named.

On April 5, 1926, von Pirquet was appointed to the League of Nations Health Service and he agreed to go to Geneva in August of that year to discuss the causes of infant mortality in the first week of life. The intensity of his activity on many health problems is evident from correspondence in the files of the League. He organized a comparative study of infant mortality in rural and urban environments which had high and low death rates, prepared what Rajchman termed "very interesting and valuable graphs" for publication in the Hygiene Committee's epidemiological report, and for the health experts he summarized data on infant mortality which had been received from various parts of the world. Although some of the representatives held differing views as to how these data should be evaluated, the lack of uniform statistics led von Pirquet to favor a clinical analysis of fatalities, with particular concern for those deaths which were avoidable. The findings were presented at an international conference on child hygiene in July, 1928, at which each delegate was asked to submit his mortality data in the form stipulated by a questionnaire. The questionnaires were then subjected to careful statistical analysis at the office of the League of Nations.

Meetings are mentioned with other delegates, one of whom was Dr. Tsurumi of Japan, who visited the *Kinderklinik*. Dr. Tsurumi was interested in nutrition, particularly in the work of the American Relief Administration and the distribution of lunches to undernourished children in the Austrian schools. In addition, von Pirquet carried on a large volume of correspondence, chiefly with Dr. Rajchman, met with him on various occasions, and suggested that a film be made to show the countryside, farms, and dwellings of Schärding in Upper Austria, one of the poorest districts in Middle Europe, in contrast with the modern children's hospitals, home for foundlings, and housing projects of Vienna. The International Health Division of the Rockefeller Foundation in Paris formally recognized von Pirquet's contributions in a letter which the secretary sent to Dr. Rajchman.

An interesting exchange of letters with Professor E. Gorter of Leyden concerned a projected conference of public health experts and pediatricians. Gorter was of the opinion that to have invitations extended by the League of Nations might cause embarrassment to the United States as a nonmember. Von Pirquet disagreed on the basis that America was already represented on the Committee for Child Hygiene.

A large amount of data on "Prohibition in Austria of the Use of Diphtheria Toxin-Antitoxin" includes a report by von Pirquet which had been approved by the Austrian Supreme Sanitary Council on January 21, 1925. It was probably based on the laboratory error previously mentioned (p. 57), in which failure to add antitoxin to vaccine resulted in the tragic death of seven infants. The subject was of great interest to American health authorities; the file contains a letter from the Massachusetts Department of Public Health. Under date of March 9, 1928, von Pirquet recommended that an organization be created by the Health Section to investigate all cases of "malignant or toxic diphtheria."

At the request of the League, he delivered two lectures in English as part of the International Continuation Course on Public Health in London. The first lecture, on November 7, 1927, dealt with tuberculosis in childhood. In the second, on November 18, he discussed practical problems of nutrition, including an explanation of his system of nutrition and of work currently being carried out in this field by his assistants.[6]

Two publications resulted from the League of Nations work. One study was based on the drastic decline in birth rate which followed the outbreak of war, causing a greater population decrease in some countries than resulted from battle casualties. Von

---

[6] "Moderne Ernährungsfragen," *Wien. med. Wchnschr.* 78 (1928): 13.

Pirquet traced the trend for more than a decade. Of the seven European belligerents, only France maintained a postwar birth level consistently above that of 1913. The greatest decline occurred among the eastern powers. Even by 1925 this trend had been only partially reversed[7] (Fig. 22). Another study showed the declining death rate between 1841 and 1920 for all but the newborn, as a result of increasing knowledge of public health.[8]

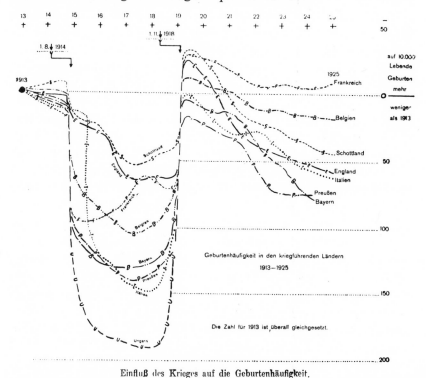

Einfluß des Krieges auf die Geburtenhäufigkeit.

Fig. 22. Influence of World War I on birth rate in Europe. *From:* "Geburtenverminderung in und nach dem Weltkriege," *Ztschr. f. soz. Hygiene "Volksgesundheit"* 1 (1927): Heft 4. (Courtesy of Urban & Schwarzenberg, Vienna.)

An article on the physical size of Austrian school children was based on almost 150,000 careful measurements taken during the feeding studies sponsored by the American Relief Administration. The figures showed that older children are heavier than younger

[7] "Geburtenverminderung in und nach dem Weltkriege," *Ztschr. f. soz. Hygiene "Volksgesundheit"* 1 (1927): Heft 4.
[8] "The Decrease of the Death Rate except among the New-Born," *Proc. Public Health Dept.*, League of Nations, 1926 (C.H./P.E. 17).

ones of the same standing or sitting height. Before puberty, boys weigh more than girls of the same height; after the onset of puberty the girls become heavier. Thus the pelidisi is higher for older than for younger children of the same sitting height. These findings confirmed Thomas Wood's law.[9] Two other publications of a statistical nature were prepared at the request of James Shotwell, secretary of the Carnegie Foundation for International Peace,[10,11] and they jointly edited a two-volume survey of public health in war. Von Pirquet engaged in other activity of a public health nature as president of the *Union Internationale de Sécours aux Enfants*.

Somewhat facetiously, von Pirquet suggested a system for designating the position of teeth in the mouth. He considered the maxilla and the mandible to be divided into two parts, represented by numerals 1 to 4 for deciduous teeth and 5 to 8 for the permanent set. A second series of numerals identified the exact location of a tooth within its quarter, numbers beginning at the center of the mouth. Thus the figure 1 was given to the central incisor, 8 to the third molar. For example, deciduous teeth in the right upper jaw are represented by the numeral 1; in the right lower jaw, numeral 3. A chart showing the entire right side of a child's mouth would combine the two digits:

$$
\begin{array}{ccccc}
15 & 14 & 13 & 12 & 11 \quad \text{(upper)} \\
\hline
35 & 34 & 33 & 32 & 31 \quad \text{(lower)}
\end{array}
$$

If the upper right canine tooth needed attention, a circle would be placed around the figure 13.[12]

Another example which characterizes the work of this period also shows clearly von Pirquet's concern for human welfare. In medicine certain concepts and procedures are carried along from one period to the next in accordance with the law of inertia. Many are eventually recognized as erroneous, but usually another generation of physicians is needed to supplant the old concept or

[9] "Anthropometrische Untersuchungen an Schulkindern in Österreich," *Ztschr. f. Kinderheilk.* 36 (1923): 63.

[10] "Ernährungszustand der Kinder in Österreich wärend des Krieges und der Nachkriegszeit," Carnegie Foundation for International Peace, 1926.

[11] "Schülerspeisung als Teil der Allgemeinen Ernährungsfürsorge. Volksgesundheit im Krieg," Carnegie Foundation for International Peace, 1926.

[12] "Nummerierung der Zähne," *Wien. klin. Wchnschr.* 23 (1924).

pseudodoxia[13] by a new one. Von Pirquet liked to apply to that phenomenon a simile taken from astronomy: "Particles emitted from rotating celestial bodies proceed in the universe in the direction of the tangent" to the sphere. Nothing can stop their course. The removal of tonsils was such a procedure.

I can still vividly remember tonsillectomy being performed without careful consideration. The surgical procedure was carried out routinely, almost as on the moving belt of a factory. When von Pirquet became director of the *Kinderklinik*, he was horrified at the routine and indiscriminate removal of tonsils, and he dealt with the problem in his characteristic way. He assigned to an intern the task of assessing the size of tonsils of a statistically significant number of normal children during each year of childhood. Analysis of figures based on 5,670 normal children disclosed a peak distribution of enlarged tonsils at the age of four years (infantile hypertrophy) and another at about the tenth year (puerile hypertrophy) (Fig. 23). Comparison showed that the peak ages for tonsillectomy at the ear, nose, and throat clinic coincided with the peaks for hypertrophy (Fig. 24). Additional information from the English statistics for 4,587 deaths from tonsillitis in the years 1911 to 1920 showed a peak of deaths at four years of age but not at ten years (Fig. 25). It thus became clear to von Pirquet that the tonsillar hypertrophy which occurred at four years and ten years of age was a physiological phenomenon which was being interfered with regardless of any real clinical necessity for surgery. After the age of ten years, natural involution of the lymphoid tissue occurs in any case.[14]

On the basis of such clear-cut findings, von Pirquet immediately discontinued routine tonsillectomy. He allowed the procedure to be carried out only when it was strongly indicated, as when the tonsils were so large that they touched in the midline and interfered with breathing and swallowing, or when there was recurrent infection of the middle ear or deafness. The policy which he advocated has become standard pediatric practice in the United States, but it was not generally accepted here until the last ten or fifteen years.

[13] Harry Bakwin, M.D., applied the term *pseudodoxia pediatrica* to the many false concepts in pediatrics.

[14] "Hypertrophia tonsillarum infantilis et puerilis," *Ztschr. f. Kinderheilk.* 39 (1925): 372.

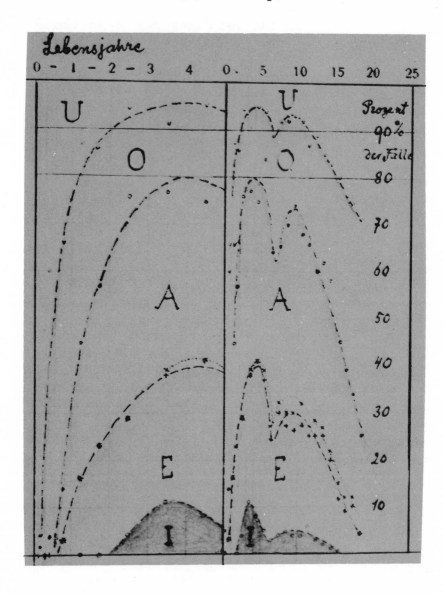

Fig. 23. Size of tonsils in 5,670 children. The first five years of age are recorded at left on an enlarged scale. Tonsil size varies from *U* (invisible) to *I* (maximum). *E*, *A*, and *O* represent intermediate sizes in descending order; $+$ = per cent of tonsillar hypertrophy; x = tonsils removed. (*Lebensjahre*—years of life; *Prozent der Fälle*—per cent of cases.) *From:* "Hypertrophia tonsillarum infantilis et puerilis," *Ztschr. f. Kinderheilk.* 39 (1925): 372. (Courtesy of Springer–Verlag, Heidelberg.)

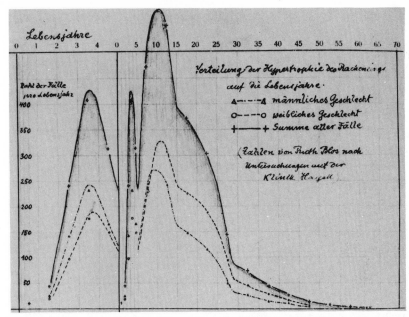

Fig. 24. Peak ages for hypertrophy of tonsils. (*Lebensjahre*—years of life; *Zahl der Fälle*—number of cases; *Verteilung der Hypertrophie des Rachenrings auf die Lebensjahre*—distribution of hypertrophy of pharyngeal ring according to age; *männliches Geschlecht*—males; *weibliches Geschlecht*—females; *Summe aller Fälle*—total cases.) From: "Hypertrophia tonsillarum infantilis et puerilis," *Ztschr. f. Kinderheilk.* 39 (1925): 374. (Courtesy of Springer–Verlag, Heidelberg.)

In this country, pseudodoxias of therapy are occasionally carried to extremes. When the concept of "focal infection" was at its most fashionable, sound teeth were pulled, the normal gall bladder or appendix was removed, and tonsillectomy was routine. The professional "tonsil snatcher" was immortalized by Sinclair Lewis in Martin Arrowsmith. Indiscriminate use of antibiotics, sulfonamides, corticosteroids, and many other drugs—not always innocuous—belongs in the same category. A common excuse is that such treatment cannot do harm. Unfortunately, however, harm sometimes *can* be done, and such therapy needs strong justification. Ideas and procedures which appear promising today may be revealed as failures tomorrow, often with far-reaching consequences. The tragically malformed infants born after their mothers had taken thalidomide is but one striking example.

The United States and Europe have basically different ideas as to the limits within which treatment is permissible and the way to educate the new generation of students. Optimism and

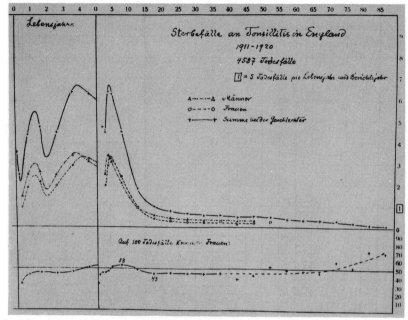

Fig. 25. 4,587 deaths from tonsillitis in England, 1911–20. ([1] = 5 deaths per year of life and of report; *Männer*—men; *Frauen*—women; *Summe beider Geschlechter*—total for both sexes; *auf 100 Todesfälle Kommen Frauen*—of 100 deaths, proportion among women.) *From:* "Hypertrophia tonsillarum infantilis et puerilis," *Ztschr. f. Kinderheilk.* 39 (1925): 377. (Courtesy of Springer-Verlag, Heidelberg.)

realism are characteristic of the American physician. He will not give in, even when the situation looks hopeless. Opening the chest in a case of cardiac arrest is not unusual. No doubt many lives have been saved or at least prolonged by the skill of the daring American surgeon. In contrast with such an optimistic outlook was the so-called "nihilistic Vienna School" of medicine. Its representatives were not reactionary, but they were conservative and skeptical, fearful to engender iatrogenic disease. Von Pirquet was of this school and in his clinical work he was always influenced by the doctrine of *primum non nocere*.

In this period he had departed almost entirely from clinical pediatrics, which no longer satisfied him. One of his British admirers, Walter R. Bett, rightly emphasized that a characteristic of Pirquet the physician was that he "never evinced deep interest in a clinical history as such."[15] He did continue his postgraduate

[15] W. R. Bett, "Some Paediatric Eponyms. I. Pirquet's Reaction," *Brit. J. Child. Dis.* 26 (1929): 276.

teaching, student lectures, and supervision of the *Kinderklinik*, although increasingly he disliked having to interrupt work in which he was engaged by the routine of a two-hour lecture to medical students. I selected the cases for presentation and, as the hour for the lecture neared, went to von Pirquet's office to review the data with him and to escort him to the lecture hall. He customarily worked in his shirt sleeves and he would put on his white coat before leaving the office. One morning he reached behind the curtain where his clothes were hanging and, instead of the hospital coat, brought out his topcoat. I waited to see what would happen and finally he realized what he was wearing. Apparently the desire for escape was strong.

Other great men similarly shifted away from their chosen fields during the final period of life. "After Newton completed the *Principia*, he suffered some sort of a 'nervous breakdown,' evidenced by increasingly unpredictable behavior. He wrote angry letters to friends and then apologized, and complained of nervous trouble and insomnia. There was a rumor that he was going out of his mind." In his last years he became interested in occult philosophy, theology, and the riddle of existence.[16] Richet, who was noted for his work on anaphylaxis, also became immersed toward the end of his life in occultism and parapsychology. Some of von Pirquet's contemporaries criticized him for abandoning pediatrics for a new field of activity. Unlike Newton or Richet, however, he remained faithful to the exact sciences. Few people followed when he penetrated into the world of numbers. His creative impulse was to reduce complex phenomena to mathematical formulae, a trend consistent with his schizothymic personality. Sometimes we are reminded of the magic square and the witches' multiplication table. The touch of magic inherent in the work of his last years is not an unusual turn in the life history of a scientist.

No one can deny that these were not the years of his greatest achievement. The creative genius of his past had burned out. Nevertheless, in his final accomplishments the mark of greatness can still be seen.

[16] "Biography of Isaac Newton," *The Sciences* (published by New York Academy of Sciences) 6 (August, 1966): 5.

XII

The Candle of Life

The seasonal incidence of mortality was not the only aspect of death which interested von Pirquet in the last years of his life. The Candle of Life, an article completed in 1929 (and submitted for publication by Edmund Nobel five years later) is concerned with the death of the individual and analyzes the hazards to which each one is subjected during his lifetime. The title refers to an Austrian superstition, and the dangers at different phases of life are compared allegorically to the manner in which a candle is consumed. A free translation follows.

The candle in the center of the Vienna birthday cake is an omen of life—the longer it burns, the more propitious the future of the birthday child. In fact, the duration of life is just as uncertain as the duration of the candle flame. At the beginning, before the candle has started to burn properly, it can be extinguished easily. Later, only a strong current of air is dangerous. At that time, however, the wick can become a robber which consumes the candle quickly, or the wick may be of poor quality in the center. Among the many candles of life, that one will shine longest which is made from the best material, whose wick burns most economically, and which has luckily escaped unfavorable circumstances.[1]

The beginnings of human life are extraordinarily dangerous. In India and China, where the tiny flame of life is not well tended, approximately half of the infants die in their first year; in the countries of northern Europe, because of better care, less than 10 out of 100 children die. This difference represents avoidable dangers and unnecessary deaths, chiefly due to nutritional disorders, infectious diseases, and inadequate care. . . .

In the second year of life the organism gradually becomes more resistant. The gusts of wind which can blow out his light of life come from the acute infectious diseases: whooping cough, measles, scarlet fever, and diphtheria. The danger from all of these diseases diminishes with increasing age. Least endangered is the child at the end of school age; the minimum number of deaths occur in the eleventh year of life. At that time even tuberculosis is almost without danger; it takes its course without clinical manifestations.

[1] All diseases can be classified simply as due to "poor make," "bad luck," or "worn out."

A few years later, however, around the age of puberty, the reaction of the organism toward the tubercle bacillus changes; the lungs are then particularly susceptible and if one does not take careful steps when the first signs of the disease are discovered, pulmonary tuberculosis can be a robber which consumes the candle of life in a few years. Girls are particularly imperiled at that time; the maximum incidence of mortality from "galloping consumption" occurs between the ages of fifteen and twenty years for the female sex. The peak for male adolescents comes a few years later. Malnutrition is especially dangerous at the time when they are beginning professional work and high physical standards are expected. In 1917, as a result of malnutrition, Vienna had its highest mortality from tuberculosis. In that year, 7,106 males died from tuberculosis, compared with 3,633 in 1913. . . .

The advent of puberty is also a peak period for deaths from such diseases as rheumatic fever, chorea, and carditis. These three diseases are related, but the causative organism is unknown and thus we do not know how to avoid them. Just as obscure is the origin of appendicitis, which also reaches its maximum in this period of life.

In unhygienic cities the most dangerous enemy of the middle-aged is typhoid fever, a disease transmitted through water. This disease diminished in Vienna from one of very frequent occurrence to a rare condition after construction of an aqueduct in the seventies of the nineteenth century.

For the female sex an enemy from another quarter now emerges: her own child. Deaths caused by the dangers of childbirth and childbed reach their climax around the thirtieth year of life.

The period from thirty to sixty years marks the onset of degenerative diseases and of chronic pulmonary tuberculosis. The lights of life in which the wick is poor or the wax of inferior quality begin to burn out. The inferior nature of the islet cells of the pancreas, for example, results in early diabetes mellitus, the inferior thyroid gland in exophthalmic goiter. Individuals weakened by syphilis come to a premature end; most deaths from general paralysis occur between forty and forty-five years, from tabes between fifty-five and sixty years. The fatal effects of alcoholism and syphilis on the liver appear between forty-five and fifty-five years. All of these conditions are chiefly dangerous for the male sex, as are the pneumonias which the aging heart can no longer cope with. Between the ages of fifty and fifty-five the maximum deaths occur from lobar pneumonia, which is twice as often fatal in males as in females. For the latter the time has come when the genitalia become susceptible to cancer (maximum between fifty and fifty-five years). Also, diseases of the veins are dangerous for them, while in the male sex the arterial system shows more rapid deterioration.

After the sixtieth year more and more candles burn down. There appear in succession cancers of the oral cavity, of the stomach, the viscera, the abdominal cavity, and finally of the skin. The cancers are true robbers; only by prompt recognition and removal can the candle of life be saved. Then follow diabetes mellitus of old age with its complications; for the male, arteriosclerosis, emphysema, and angina pectoris; for the female, chronic rheumatoid disease, embolism, and thrombosis.

After the eightieth year of life only those candles remain burning which had good wicks and good wax and were not reached by a gust of wind. Now the brain can quit working and succumb to a hemorrhage, or senile gangrene may occur. Finally only a tiny stump remains which is weakened to such a degree that it may succumb to any current of air. A slight pulmonary infection or intestinal disorder blows out the tiny light just as easily as the newly lighted candle of life of the newborn. . . .

In the last eighty years Europeans have made great progress in regard to life expectation: only half as many candles of life go out on lighting; the gusts of wind which in later childhood blow out the light of life are diminished to one third. The robbers which steal the years of manhood have been weakened by the progress of medicine and surgery; and even the candle stumps of old age are better cared for. However, we have not yet progressed so far as to provide the candle of life with a better wick, to renew its wax, or to restore the whole candle from broken pieces.[2]

This unique example of von Pirquet's reasoning, unaccompanied by charts, was found in his desk after his death. The manuscript was in handwritten form and evidently he had not tried to publish it. However, he once showed it to me, and expressed pleasure with the allegory he had built around the candle in the center of the child's birthday cake. In enumerating just before his own death the dangers encountered during the whole life span, he may have had in mind an idea similar to Robert Browning's "last of life for which the first was made."

[2] "Die Lebenskerze," *Wien. med. Wchnschr.* 84 (1934): 537. (Courtesy of Verlag Brüder Hollinek, Vienna.)

XIII

Allergy of the Life Phases

Just as the research which established von Pirquet's reputation dealt with the theory of allergy, so too his last work was concerned with the same subject, although viewed from a somewhat different aspect which widened its original meaning. In his own words, it was the opening up of unexplored regions of biology and medicine. When von Pirquet coined the term allergy in 1906 he was contemplating the changed state of an organism produced through accidental contact or purposeful treatment with certain foreign agents, the tacit assumption being that the individual organism was otherwise unaltered. In his last years he was occupied with the problem of how far the reaction toward disease is conditioned by spontaneous changes taking place within the organism itself during its life course rather than by any treatment it had previously undergone.

Von Pirquet first became interested in this subject in 1915. The introduction to his monograph on malignant tumors explains that he then noticed how many more girls than boys (up to the age of fourteen) were admitted to the tuberculosis ward on the flat roof of the *Kinderklinik*. The observation suggested that, before the age of fourteen, fewer boys than girls had pulmonary tuberculosis. Such a medico-statistical problem always appealed to him and he obtained further data from the vital statistics for England and Wales. He pursued the subject throughout his life, and his guiding thought was expressed as follows:

Almost every well-defined cause of death has its characteristic age curve. Even in infectious diseases the previously accepted idea that the causative organism represents the main factor is not correct; the second, usually more essential, factor is the sensitivity of the individual and this in turn is primarily a sensitivity related to age.[1]

Originally he had intended to publish a complete atlas showing the age of distribution for diseases but, through his zeal in pursuing

[1] *Die Allergie des Lebensalters. Die Bösartigen Geschwülste* (Leipzig: Georg Thieme, 1930).

187

any point which especially interested him, more and more data were accumulated. At the time of his death the atlas was not complete, although the age distribution for a few diseases had been summarized[2] (Fig. 26).

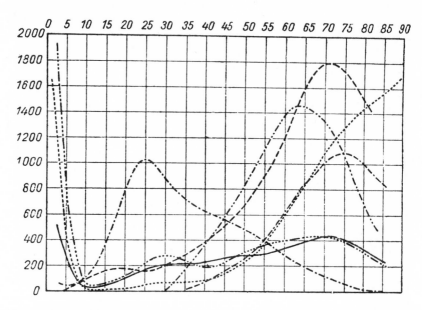

Fig. 26. Number of deaths from major diseases. (Vertical scale—Deaths per year; Horizontal scale—Years of life.)

———————	Influenza	— — — — —	Malignant tumors
—·—·—·—·—	Pulmonary tuberculosis	··········	Bronchitis
—··—··—	Cancer	—······—	Pneumonia
— — ·— — ·	Cerebral hemorrhage		

From: "Allergie des Lebensalters," *Wien. klin. Wchnschr.* 42 (1929): 65. (Courtesy of Springer-Verlag, Heidelberg.)

Tuberculosis. When the British mortality statistics were plotted graphically, the rising curve for deaths from pulmonary tuberculosis occurred several years later in boys than in girls. Von Pirquet noticed that the curve had two peaks, one in the first year of life and the second at about the twentieth year, separated by a depression. The first peak represented the manifestations of disseminated tuberculosis, such as meningitis, tuberculosis of the bones, miliary tuberculosis, and primary tuberculosis of the lungs. The incidence of these forms decreased from year to year; not

[2] "Allergie des Lebensalters," *Wien. klin. Wchnschr.* 42 (1929): 65.

until puberty did pulmonary tuberculosis of the adult type emerge in either sex as a new form of the disease. Its earlier onset in girls was attributed to their attainment of sexual maturity at a younger age. At puberty a change occurs in the body reaction to the tubercle bacillus, which von Pirquet had noted in his primary concept of allergy. He compared it with the altered reactions of the skin toward tuberculin.

Apart from the influence of puberty, he found no marked effect of sex on the mortality curve of tuberculosis. The profound influence of age of onset on the curve was equal in both sexes. The first signs of human infection seem to be much the same at all ages. The primary infection, the Ghon tubercle, for instance, and the behavior of the regional lymph nodes show no essential difference at this stage. The secondary stage, however, which comes soon after, is strongly influenced by age in its behavior and its extension in time and space. The infant tends to get a secondary dissemination of tubercles which by preschool age is restricted chiefly to the surface of the body; by school age a secondary spread does not usually take place. The influence of age is shown even more clearly at the tertiary stage, with the development of lung cavities in undernourished adolescents who had a primary infection in early childhood. The peak in the death rate between the ages of fifteen and twenty-five, von Pirquet called the specific "allergy of age" for tuberculosis.

At one time Egon Helmreich, a junior staff member of the *Kinderklinik,* wrote a paper on tuberculosis. All manuscripts published by the staff had first to be approved by von Pirquet, and the usual procedure was for the young man to read his paper aloud. Helmreich had stated, in contradiction of von Pirquet's teaching, that pulmonary tuberculosis in adolescence was a new infection, unrelated to the previous stages of the disease. When the reading was finished von Pirquet said: "My dear Sir, in my clinic this is heresy. You may publish the paper if you wish, but you will have to add a footnote stating that you do so against the advice of your chief." Helmreich deleted the offending portion before he submitted the article for publication.

Syphilis. The allergy of age can be clearly observed in the mortality curves for general paralysis and tabes. Here, too, the primary infection is probably not greatly influenced by the age at onset, but in the tertiary stage the effects on the brain and spinal cord are associated with a specific change in nerve tissues associated with age. Deaths from general paralysis rise steeply at about the thirtieth year of life and reach their peak at the forty-third year; a steep decline then follows. It is probably because of sensitivity that only 15 to 20 per cent of all cases of general paralysis occur in the female sex, since it is unlikely that five times as many men as women should acquire syphilis. In tabes, on the other hand, the peak of mortality does not occur until the age of fifty-seven. Here again, a special allergy of the central nervous system at a certain age must be responsible.

Diabetes. A sharply defined age distribution is seen not only in the degenerative diseases, attributable to bacterial or bacterio-toxic agents, but also in metabolic diseases such as diabetes melli-tus which are related to hereditary weakness. The mortality curve in groups over the age of forty (Fig. 27) shows an increasing

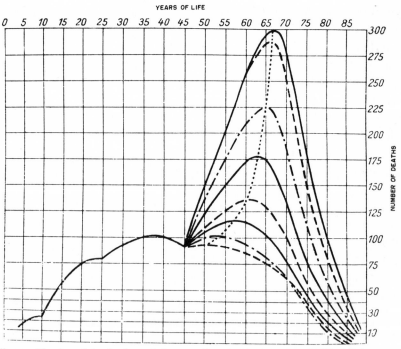

Fig. 27. Number of deaths from diabetes mellitus in England and Wales, 1848 to 1920. The eight curves represent, respectively (reading from bottom to top of chart), the calendar years 1848–54, 1855–60, 1861–70, 1871–80, 1881–90, 1891–1900, 1901–10, 1911–20. The vertical dotted line, or axis of symmetry, goes through the peak for each curve. Von Pirquet took as a base line 100 deaths at age forty and worked out comparative ratios for subsequent ages. *From:* "Allergie des Lebensalters," *Wien. klin. Wchnschr.* 42 (1929): 65. (Courtesy of Springer–Verlag, Heidelberg.)

number of deaths from the diabetes of old age. The curve begins to rise in the forty-fourth year of life and reaches its peak in the seventh decade. Von Pirquet's data showed that the number of deaths from senile diabetes had 'increased progressively for the previous ninety years.

The significance of his chart was confirmed by the report of a recent conference of the New York Academy of Sciences at which two different types of diabetes mellitus were discussed. Refined biochemical procedures have shown that pancreatic deficiency is responsible for only 20 per cent of diabetes mellitus. This group of patients, known as "growth-onset" or juvenile diabetics, depend on treatment with insulin. In contrast, the "maturity-onset" type of diabetes which begins after the age of forty can often be controlled without insulin.[3]

Cirrhosis of the Liver. In cirrhosis the findings are remarkably similar. The mortality curve rises in the fourth decade, has a sharp maximum at about fifty-five years, then a rapid decline. Cirrhosis of the liver is predominantly a disease of males. As in many other diseases, the peak occurs five years earlier in females.

Rheumatic Process. Particularly remarkable is the allergy of the life phases in the rheumatic diseases. Chorea and acute rheumatic fever are diseases of youth. Their mortality peak occurs between the ages of ten and fifteen years; however, the curves do not rise from birth, but begin at the end of the third year of life. Von Pirquet speculated whether they might not be secondary mani-festations, analogous with tuberculosis and syphilis: "Is the organism during the first three years of life not able to contract the infection, or is it simply unable to produce secondary mani-festations? One may speculate that the primary infection (hith-erto entirely unknown) might be acquired at any time in child-hood, but that a tendency to secondary manifestations occurs only in a certain period."[4]

[3] "Conference on Diabetes and Obesity," *The Sciences* (published by New York Academy of Sciences) 7 (June, 1967): 12.

[4] Current medical thinking assumes a latent period between the primary infection and the appearance of actual (secondary) clinical signs, which are now regarded as the expression of an allergic state. The hemolytic Streptococcus is considered to be the primary infective agent which sensitizes the organism to produce clinical signs of rheumatic fever. What can be observed is actually an antigen-antibody reaction in the fullest sense understood by von Pirquet, but the resistance of the organism to rheumatic fever in the first three years of life is still not explained.

Von Pirquet called attention to another remarkable fact, namely, that the incidence of appendicitis, the genesis of which is unknown, is closely related to the incidence of the rheumatic complex. The curves for the rheumatic diseases and for appendicitis (Fig. 28) show that chronic rheumatism has the characteristics of an entirely different disease. The acute process reaches its peak between the ages of ten and fifteen years, whereas the curve for the chronic process rises between the ages of forty and sixty and reaches its maximum after the seventieth year of life. This group of diseases is obviously not homogeneous.

Malignant Tumors. In his introduction to the monograph on the allergies of the life phases for malignant tumors, von Pirquet states: "Every physician knows that malignant tumors are diseases of old age, but this general recognition is often blotted from our memory by the cases of juvenile malignancy. They are so exceptional that they stand out vividly in our minds." The number of deaths before the thirtieth year is very small, but the curve then rises steeply and continuously to a peak in the sixty-fifth year. Each kind of malignant growth has its characteristic peak.

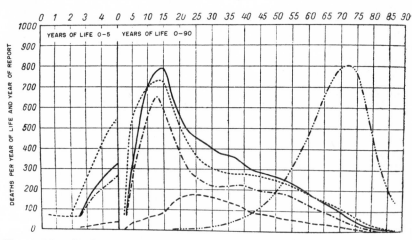

Fig. 28. Mortality from the rheumatic diseases.
—————— Total from chorea, rheumatic fever, and endocarditis
— · — · —· Rheumatic fever
· · · · · · · · · · Endocarditis
— — — — Appendicitis
— · · · — · · · Chronic rheumatism
From: "Allergie des Lebensalters," *Wien. klin. Wchnschr.* 42 (1929): 65. (Courtesy of Springer–Verlag, Heidelberg.)

The statistics for internal diseases are unreliable inasmuch as they are affected markedly by changes in diagnostic terminology. In some diseases, changes of medical opinion can be inferred from the figures, but diagnosis of malignant tumors has not changed for many decades. A cancer of the lip, tongue, rectum, or breast is quite unmistakable. The malignant tumors of internal organs are less utilizable from individual figures, but here also the statistics are extraordinarily consistent, favoring the homogeneity of the disease as well as the reliability of the diagnosis.

The causes for the differing age distributions of allergies, about which von Pirquet speculated, cannot be identified yet. In pulmonary tuberculosis it may be justifiable to think that susceptibility to the disease in the years of puberty is in some way related to the gonads. "It appears probable that endocrinology and genetics will explain a good deal of the phenomena . . . but we are still busy collecting facts to point the way into unexplored areas of medicine."

This final, somewhat mysterious, book was feverishly produced during the last days of his life. The allergy of the life phases for malignant growths is the only portion of the projected atlas which was completed and this was published as a separate monograph. In his last lecture to the students von Pirquet discussed the conclusions of the book. An artistic table summarized his interpretation of the vital statistics.

With this return to the doctrine of allergy his life work was completed and the ring closed.

XIV

The Suicide

On February 28, 1929, Clemens von Pirquet and his wife were found dead. The verdict at the inquest was suicide by cyanide poisoning. A premonitory episode which occurred a few years earlier may shed light on von Pirquet's state of mind. In 1925, when he was president of the *Deutsche Gesellschaft für Kinderheilkunde,* he and Maria arrived in Karlsbad, Czechoslovakia, on the afternoon before the opening session. Everyone observed that he was in good spirits as he went for a walk with his friends von Gröer, Nobel, and Wagner. Meanwhile, at the hotel Madame von Pirquet complained that the room reserved for them on the fourth floor was unsuitable; she had already compared it with a more attractive room assigned to another prominent member of the congress. Their room was exchanged for one on the second floor, and that circumstance may have saved her husband's life.

In the evening he went to bed early because of a slight cold, and took a sleeping pill so as to be in good condition for delivering the opening address the next day. At two o'clock in the morning he jumped from the window. He landed on his feet, with no injury other than fractures of both calcanei. During the incident Madame von Pirquet remained in deep sleep under the influence of her nightly dose of Veronal. The fractures were competently treated by an orthopedic surgeon who was one of the guest speakers at the meeting, but the news of the accident had profoundly shocked and subdued the delegates.

On the following morning von Pirquet offered an interesting explanation. He said he had dreamed that he was locked in a burning sheep barn, and in his dream had jumped from the window in order to save himself. He was his usual collected self, not depressed, and even made one of his witty, cynical remarks in which he compared the sheep in the barn with the pediatricians assembled at the meeting. Everybody was happy that he seemed himself again. His explanation still leaves unanswered the question: Did the accident result from the slight infection and from an abnormal reaction to the drug? He had never before taken a barbiturate.

Be that as it may, in the age of Freud and of the association of dreams with the unconscious it did not require much imagination to interpret the accident as an unconscious attempt at suicide. The psychoanalyst who expressed that opinion in an interview given to one of the Viennese newspapers certainly welcomed it as an explanation. What the analyst did not then recognize as important, however, was that Clemens' wife was left behind. The actual suicide three-and-a-half years later was of a different nature. It had been carefully premeditated but must have been linked with the previous unconscious attempt. Although the premeditation subsequently became increasingly clear, none of us who were his immediate associates had any prior inkling that he might commit suicide. When the distressing news reached the *Kinderklinik* late at night that von Pirquet and Maria were both dead there was almost universal disbelief. The events of that night of February 28, 1929, are as sharply alive in my mind as though the tragedy had happened yesterday.

Why? Why should a man of von Pirquet's intellectual stature, at the age of fifty-five, at the summit of a successful career, admired by the world and beloved by his friends and colleagues, decide to end his life? He had tried hard, although unsuccessfully, to conceal the real nature of his death and to make it appear an accident. In the morning he had phoned the hospital to report that the gas heater in his bathroom had been leaking and, as a result of the escaping carbon monoxide, he did not feel well and would stay at home. In the afternoon he invited Dr. Edmund Nobel, his first assistant and friend, to come for a short visit. Nobel left without being aware that anything abnormal was impending. The adopted children were away at that time. In the evening a niece who was staying with the von Pirquets attended the theater with their housekeeper. During that interval without interruption, which undoubtedly had been arranged as part of the suicide plan, the couple took potassium cyanide and ended their lives. The bottle which contained the poison was later found in their room. It had been obtained on prescription only two days before as part of an order for several disinfectants to be used in the stable of his estate and was supplied by the pharmacist without question.

One can still speculate about the motive. There was no explanation in von Pirquet's will and no admission that suicide was intended. Many factors obviously worked together. Yet one thing is certain—he was at the end of his resources and was unwilling to continue a life which no longer offered anything which he found attractive or appealing. All previous attempts at solving his problems must have failed.

It is of little avail to look at the catastrophe from a psychiatric point of view. There are moments when death has no terrors but is a deliverance from hardship and insoluble conflict. It is too simple to resort to the Freudian death urge as an explanation. The concept of a *Todestrieb* which drives every individual to pursue his life course, with death and the consequent return to the inorganic as the ultimate aim, may be farfetched. Yet a *Todestrieb* is a genuine attitude of mind in some aging people who feel that their powers are failing and it is time to go. This attitude is present most notably, of course, in the minds of suicides and of the very many "normal" people to whom the impulse to commit suicide is familiar but who never reach the point of carrying it out. Perhaps most often suicide appears as the only means of ultimate escape from the strains and stresses of a world that has become unbearable. Sometimes it may be a self-inflicted punishment for guilt. Here Freud is probably right in calling it an act of aggression directed against oneself.

Freud also compared the unyielding pursuit of an idea by the great discoverers and inventors with the *idée fixe* of compulsory neurotics. Examples are the use of cocaine as an anesthetic in the eye, proposed by Koller, and Robert Meyer's law of the preservation of energy. If the new idea is rejected, the discoverer may have a monomaniacal urge to defend it to his last breath. Some individuals escape into overt insanity (Semmelweis and Meyer ended in asylums) or commit suicide. When von Pirquet proposed his new system of nutrition the pattern was similar. Strong opposition arose from both contemporary pediatricians and physiologists, yet he never gave in. Whether his suicide was related to this opposition is pure speculation.

The strikingly uneven character of von Pirquet's creative activity has been pointed out: Periods of intensive creativeness alternated with periods of nonproductivity. This phenomenon, certain strange ·ˈ which appeared in his later work, and the choice of a severely psychoneurotic marital companion (to whom he remained devoted with touching faithfulness) make one suspect the presence of neurotic reactions. Did such reactions first fan the fire of his intellect and later unhinge his mind? In the first Vienna period of creativeness, von Pirquet's genius expanded freely and fruitfully. Later appeared the tendency to surround his thinking with rules, schemes and systems, sober figures, and constraining formulas and equations—all foreign to and cramping the mind of a genius. Was this tendency in part buried in a deep impulse, in part called upon to keep a tight rein on the escaping inner striving? We do not know. However, we do know that we owe a great debt of gratitude to this man for his far-reaching and fruitful activity.

The chronic, incurable ailment of his wife, frictions and a lawsuit within his own family with attendant newspaper publicity may have been contributory factors during a phase when von Pirquet's mental activity was at a low ebb, but they cannot be considered the real cause. His was not a depressive personality. The suicide decision was made deliberately, weeks in advance, like other important decisions in his life. He was always afraid of becoming senile, and many sarcastic remarks that he made about aging members of the faculty are remembered. Some of his contemporaries and relatives blamed Maria as the instigator, but theirs were only vague speculations; the exact emotional sequence remains a mystery.

Looking back after more than thirty-five years since his tragic death, we may ask whether mankind might have expected more from him if his life and work had not been interrupted. We may answer with Nietzsche: Everybody dies at the right time. Goethe once expressed a similar belief when engaged in a conversation with Eckermann which turned to the subject of early death:

Do you know how I see it? Man must be brought to naught again. Every exceptional person has a certain mission he is called upon to fulfil. When he has accomplished it, he is no longer needed on earth in this form, and providence makes use of him again for something else. But since here below everything happens in a natural way, the demons trip him up over and over again until finally he succumbs. Thus it was with Napoleon and many others. Mozart died in his thirty-sixth year, Raphael at about the same age, and Byron was only a little older. But all had fulfilled their missions consummately, and it was probably time for them to go, so that something should remain for other people to do in the long destined duration of this world's existence.[1]

The curve of von Pirquet's productivity showed a steep ascent in his youthful years, a long level period of maturity and of harvesting what he had sown, and a slow but definite decline as he approached his fiftieth year. Like other geniuses, he reached the summit of his creative activity at about the age of thirty.

A few days after his death an oil painting which he had ordered was delivered to Nobel. It showed a blasted tree struck by lightning. That von Pirquet was spared from becoming nonproductive and senile helps to reconcile us to the tragedy of his self-inflicted death. If he had lived until the coming of Hitler, he would have been humiliated and deprived of his official position as professor of pediatrics at the University, since his ancestry did not include the minimum requirement of Aryan grandparents.

The newspapers expanded upon the suicide in big headlines. Gossip and rumor flourished. One paper grossly distorted the scarcely known facts and indulged in fantastic interpretations which lacked any tangible foundation. It is completely incorrect that his wife made him a drug addict; it is also incorrect that he suffered from depression. Although the illness of his wife often interrupted his daily activities, she did not interfere in any important way with his duties as head of the department of pediatrics or with his research activities, and he achieved the goals which he considered of greatest importance.

On the afternoon of the day before his suicide he went to a meeting of the *Union Internationale de Sécours aux Enfants* (U.I.S.E.) in the *Kinderklinik*, addressed a group of high-school girls, and distributed awards for sketches best illustrating the principles of the U.I.S.E. He was as calm as usual and in his best humor as he talked to the girls. Afterward he attended a faculty meeting and nominated Dr. Lazar, one of his assistants, for the rank of professor. It is pure press conjecture that doubts as to the soundness of his scientific work had entered his mind and made him an easy prey to his wife's persuasion to commit suicide. It is incorrect that antagonism between the Austrian and the North German schools of pediatrics, or more specifically between

[1] *Goethe: His Life and Times*, transl. Richard Friedenthal (Cleveland: World Publishing Co., 1965), p. 26. (Courtesy of The World Publishing Company, Cleveland.)

Vienna and Berlin, contributed to the crisis or that the rejection of some of his theories of nutrition had depressed him. It is true that there were antagonisms and controversies, but that is not unusual in scientific discussions. There was no ill feeling, and von Pirquet's personality did not suffer from an inferiority complex.

The last meeting of the German Pediatric Society which he attended was that held in 1928 in Hamburg. He left Hamburg soon after he had delivered his speech, without waiting for the banquet, not because of criticism but because he went with his wife to Hanover to visit her relatives. During the meeting she had spent the days in bed and he remained with her most of the time. His absence may have given the impression that he had withdrawn from the crowd; however, those who were familiar with his behavior in similar situations knew that it was not unusual.

In von Pirquet's last will, written shortly before his death, one paragraph is directed to the medical faculty of the University. He asked them to nominate one of his pupils as his successor.

My *Klinik* is a complicated organism; its functioning is built upon my personal innovations. Someone who does not understand the management, and who would try to change to another scientific system, would destroy the advantages of the *Klinik*. The following of my pupils (in alphabetical order) are able to succeed me: Franz von Gröer, Ernst Mayerhofer, Edmund Nobel, Bela Schick, Richard Wagner, Hans Wimberger.

None of them was chosen. The faculty appointed as his successor Franz Hamburger, a professor of pediatrics from one of the provincial universities of Austria, who had his own ideas and transplanted his own staff to Vienna. And so a glorious period of Viennese pediatrics came to an end.

In his last letter, written in pencil to Nobel on the day of the suicide, von Pirquet still tried to conceal his intentions. Quite casually he mentioned that he usually made careful preparation before going on a trip to have his affairs in order in the event of sudden death;[2] he did so that particular night because he could not sleep. He advised Nobel to approach the mayor of the city of Vienna and request a grave of honor in the cemetery. He was

[2] He was expected to go to Berlin to accept the Aronson Prize, one of the highest German awards in bacteriology.

so sure of his greatness that he did not hesitate to make that demand. Should his wife die at the same time, he wanted her buried in the same grave. He said he would prefer that no autopsies be made; nobody would have an interest in the outcome since their lives were not insured.

After the disclosure of suicide the Catholic Church was prepared to deny the von Pirquets a Christian burial, but the Dean of the Medical Faculty intervened with the Archbishop and the suicides were declared to have been committed while in a state of mental imbalance. To many that may appear an insignificant formality, but it is the view of the Church that suicide carried out in a lucid state of mind is sinful, or at least a violation of one's duty to society and oneself. What exactly are one's duties to oneself it is difficult to determine. Nature has bestowed upon man alone the prerogative of terminating his own life, in contrast with the animals whose urge it is to live as long as possible. The animal is exposed solely to the physical afflictions of the present, but the human is exposed to mental sufferings derived from the past and the future as well. A permanent state of discomfort can produce weariness with life, and a quite insignificant trouble can tip the balance. Von Pirquet was obviously in such a state of mind when he committed suicide with cool deliberation and firm purpose. It is hard to see him as a sick man or to interpret his suicide as a product of mental illness. On the contrary, he remains in memory as a healthy, sound person who terminated his life at his own convenience.

> Vainly the gale will shake the withered oak,
> But with a crash he flings the living down,
> Grasping with ruffian hands her copious locks.[3]

Two years after his death a monument on the grave and a bust in front of the *Kinderklinik* were unveiled, and the city of Vienna named a great block of flats in one of its housing estates after him. While he was still alive, a street in a small village near Vienna had been named *Dr. Clemens Pirquetgasse*. More than thirty years after his death an international committee was

---

[3] Heinrich von Kleist, *Penthesilea*. The Classic Theatre, ed. Eric R. Bentley; transl. Humphry Trevelyan (Toronto: Doubleday & Co., 1959). (Courtesy of Doubleday Publishers, Toronto.)

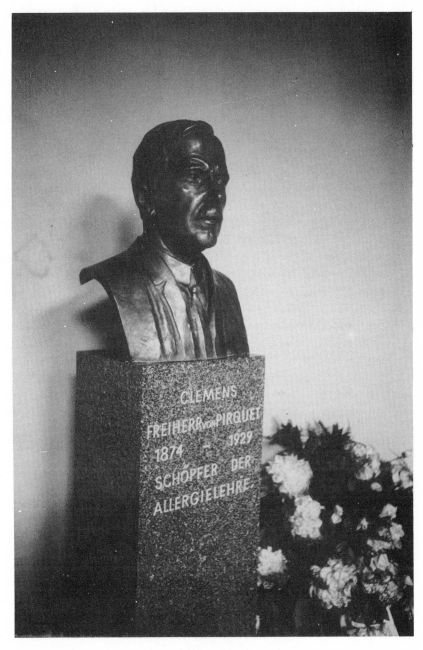

Bust of von Pirquet at University of Vienna.
(Courtesy of Black Star Publishing Co., New York City.)

established in Boston to raise the Clemens von Pirquet Memorial Fund for erecting a memorial in the arcaded quadrangle of the University of Vienna where the great men of Vienna medicine are remembered. A bust of von Pirquet was unveiled there by the Rector of the University on October 23, 1962, in the presence of a distinguished company.

XV

Final Chapter

All great advances in medicine are related to a specific environment, an auspicious period in time, and a given subject. Nevertheless, even under these circumstances an outstanding mind is needed to grasp the essential principles and use them to initiate scientific progress. Von Pirquet had such a mind; his early work started a trend in medical science which is still continuing.

An international atmosphere for immune-biological research had been established at the beginning of the century by von Behring, Ehrlich, Bordet, and Richet. In Vienna the leaders were Max Gruber and Rudolf Kraus; Escherich's clinic provided the environment for pediatric research. Against this background, in rapid succession, came von Pirquet's discoveries in serum sickness (1905), vaccination and vaccinial allergy (1907), the cutaneous effect of tuberculin (1908), and the general mechanism of allergy. These studies were all variations of the same theme. Light was shed on the pathological processes and reactions within the body and its deep-seated tissues when the scientific observer saw the changeable pattern on the skin as evidence of the state of internal organs. The previously sealed book of nature opened to one able to decipher its strange hieroglyphics. The use of harmless or even beneficial "poisons" permitted safe clinical experimentation and a wide variation of experimental conditions. Animal experiments, about which von Pirquet had always been skeptical, could be eliminated.

Even in his early observations one may recognize the methods which led to his success: subtle observation at the bedside and graphic representation of all findings, even those hitherto overlooked or apparently meaningless; correlation of such findings with the causes and course of illness; thoughtful study of all signs and symptoms, logically and in sequence, in anticipation of the final outcome. In this way an abundance of data was collected. The secondary, delayed toxic effects of horse serum, unlike the familiar primary toxic effects of various other substances, were interpreted as an antibody response. The period of time after the injection until antibodies are formed is the measure of the delayed action. This can be recognized through the phenomenon of an accelerated or immediate reaction in an individual whose body defenses are increased by previous invasion of the same causative organism. If inanimate toxins act only after a definite incubation period, then in infectious disease the incubation is not solely the period required for the causative organism to produce a given level of toxin. A function inherent in the host must also enter into the equation.

Briefly, this is the Pirquet-Schick theory of incubation time. The pathogenic agent causes symptoms of illness in the organism only when modified by antibodies; incubation time is the period which elapses prior to the formation of antibodies. Von Pirquet considered the onset of signs of illness, not their termination, an indication of antibody formation. The shortened incubation time following a second injection of horse serum suggested to him that serum sickness was induced by the collision of *antigen and antibodies*. The earlier the reaction of the organism and the less time the foreign intruder has had to propagate, the faster its development is inhibited and the milder is the injury inflicted. Thus becomes evident the teleological significance of accelerated defense in infections and the lasting resistance acquired when an individual suffers a primary disease. This protection was originally thought to be a humoral immunity or insensitiveness; at present it is interpreted as cellular hypersensitivity. The notion of immunity was carried over from the time when hypersensitivity was unknown, and the two can be closely related even though the words are contradictory. Immunology was in need of a term to characterize an organism's ability to react with any toxin, live or inanimate. For this general concept, von Pirquet offered the term *allergy*.

He did not discover new territory, but created ideas and concepts. Like the great masters of the fine arts, he selected not *rare* but *old*, much-studied problems and successfully reshaped them. The adverse effects of horse serum and the course of vaccination were well known, but out of confusing data von Pirquet crystallized new concepts of serum sickness, incubation time, and allergy. Knowledge of vaccination was advanced far more in a few months than in decades before. A procedure known since

Jenner, demonstrated to the physician a thousand times a year and supposedly well understood, was placed in new light. Von Pirquet interpreted the interaction between host and pathogen clearly, without confusing details.

Vivid feeling for the help which suffering mankind expects of the medical profession prevented him from losing himself in basic research. He was determined to link science with the demands of the day. In addition, he was successful in stimulating his pupils and contemporaries into a consideration of the needs of the future. His contributions in the field of tuberculosis will not be forgotten. By means of the diagnostic test named for him the internal tuberculous process could be interpreted from a reaction on the surface of the skin, even though the focus might be too small for detection by physical examination or X-ray. The significance of the tuberculin test for estimating the incidence of the disease, for detecting contacts, for social welfare, and indirectly for preventing tuberculosis is too far-reaching for brief discussion. Worried parents whose child had been taken to sanatoria for many years because of weight loss, slightly elevated temperature, cough, joint pains, or enlargement of the cervical lymph nodes might now be told with certainty that the cause was not tuberculosis. This was von Pirquet's gift to the medical profession and to mankind.

Von Pirquet may rightly be called the father of diagnostic skin testing. Numerous modifications of his tuberculin test were later introduced. The concept was applied to other diseases as cutaneous and intracutaneous diagnostic tests were developed for smallpox, leprosy, trichophytosis, actinomycosis, syphilis, glanders, Echinococcus infestation, trichinosis, and cat-scratch fever. It also was the basis for the diphtheria test of Schick.

Not only did von Pirquet himself have an appreciation for calculations, graphic analysis, and statistical interpretation, but he awakened a similar interest among his professional colleagues. He applied these methods in an ingenious experiment to popularize the science of nutrition. Even though the forces involved cannot be expressed in a simple formula, and a scientific system for general use can hardly be obtained, through his efforts a large segment of the population was taught careful utilization of food.

It may still be too soon to appreciate the full significance of his scientific accomplishments and his contributions to pediatrics and the broader field of medical thinking. A full evaluation of his activities must be left to history. Even the first period of his work is still influencing medical thought. The concept of allergy, which was the forerunner for total biologic-medical research, is even now gaining in importance. An ingeniously devised and masterfully handled theory led to the characterization of serum sickness, clarification of the essence of vaccinial allergy, establishment of the concept of allergy, the theory of incubation, and finally the discovery of the cutaneous tuberculin test. Von Pirquet was both a creative thinker and a clinical observer who knew how to analyze clinical data by graphic procedures. From simple clinical phenomena came a fund of new ideas which previous generations had neglected.

The same outstanding productive qualities distinguished von Pirquet as organizer and leader of his Vienna clinic. The spirit and the individuality of the world-renowned *Kinderklinik* resulted from its harmonious union of research institute, model hospital, educational facility, and intellectual center for social welfare. The scientific trend of the organization gave free play to the individual development of von Pirquet's pupils. Hence his inner staff, in spite of their close relationship, never developed into a cult.

Care for the well-being of the child was the first concern of the *Kinderklinik*. Its organization was such that the most minute clinical details were easily accessible and could be scientifically utilized by any physician. The nursing staff had an established reputation which was admired even in countries like England and the United States which had had long experience in modern nursing techniques. Von Pirquet was active in furthering the development of a well-trained, intelligent staff of nurses with outstanding ethical and scientific qualifications. In addition to painstaking attention to perfecting their working skills, he introduced new methods of clinical observation, and nurses were taught to record clinical data according to his graphic method. As a result a unique, highly disciplined group was created which made possible the realization of von Pirquet's ambitious clinical experiments.

His subtle social perception imbued his *Klinik* with the spirit of social medicine at a time when this trend had not developed in children's hospitals. In an atmosphere which emphasized child welfare, the socio-medical thinking of physicians, nurses, and students who received training there was stimulated. Innovations consistent with this attitude were the first psychiatric ward for children; a preventorium for tuberculosis; an open-air ward in the midst of a city for children with latent tuberculosis; well-baby clinics; and the training of hosts of social workers. Von Pirquet's other social activities included the founding of an Austrian society of public health, and his service as president of the *Union Internationale de Sécours aux Enfants* and as chairman of the Committee for Child Hygiene of the League of Nations.

Evidences of his position of esteem were shown by the fact that he was the subject of two doctoral theses, one written in Germany and the other in Holland.[1,2] In New York City a Von Pirquet Society of Clinical Medicine was formed in 1964, which holds frequent meetings.

In public and in private life, as teacher, leader, friend, and colleague, Clemens von Pirquet distinguished himself by his charm, unlimited kindness, and tact (or what one of his witty colleagues called *Clementia praecox*). The nobility of his character and the depth of his culture attracted everyone with whom he came in contact. Firm determination, seriousness, and sympathy were combined in the noted physician, scientist, and humanitarian who furthered the high ideals of western civilization by banishing *hate* and placing *love* first in his struggle to alleviate the sufferings of mankind.

[1] W. Huitema, *Clemens Pirquet* (Amsterdam: Jacob van Campen, 1936).
[2] Elsbeth Hoff, *Das Leben und Wirken des Wiener Klinikers Clemens Freiherr v. Pirquet* (Düsseldorf: G. H. Nolte, 1937).

INDEX

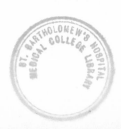

Designed by Edward D. King
Composed in 11 on 13 Caslon Old Style by
Baltimore Type and Composition Corp.
Printed offset by Universal Lithographers, Inc. on P & S, R.
Bound by L. H. Jenkins in Arrestox 15260
with Slate blue, multicolor endpapers
Jacket printed in two colors by John D. Lucas Printing Company

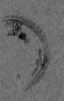